Createspace Publishing
Printed in United States

Book formatting: bookclaw.com

ISBN 13: 9781925792300

Disclaimer
Note well that the information provided in this book is designed to provide helpful and common-sense type information on the subjects discussed. They are insights and experiences from my life experience only. This book is not meant to be used, nor should it be used, to diagnose or treat any medical condition. For diagnosis and/or proper treatment of any medical/emotional of physical problems, it is imperative you consult with a reputable professional physician/therapist. Please be advised that as the reader you are responsible for your own decisions, actions, and resulting outcomes.

"My Body is Mine, Not Yours!" (Part 2) is a handbook written to be used in a responsible manner with the supervision of a qualified counsellor, healthcare professional and/or caregiver. "My Body Is Mine, Not Yours!" is highly recommended to be utilised in conjunction with "The 3 E's Caregivers and Educators Instructional Companion Guide" (Part 1).

Please Note: A percentage of all sales are charitably donated to assist in the education and prevention of child sexual abuse and Suicide Prevention Australia to assist in the prevention of suicide.

Ordering Information
For quantities; special discounts are available on quantity purchases by corporations, schools, associations, and others.

Contact Details:
Website: www.njlutter.com

The 3 E's

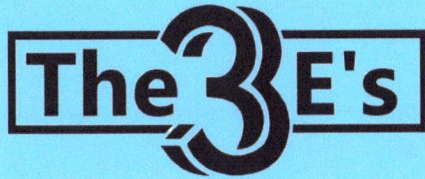

Please see "My Body Is Mine, Not Yours!"
the accompanying (Part 1) guide

Caregivers and Educators
Companion Instructional Guide

"My Body Is Mine, Not Yours!"

N J Lutter

"My Body Is Mine, Not Yours!"

N J Lutter

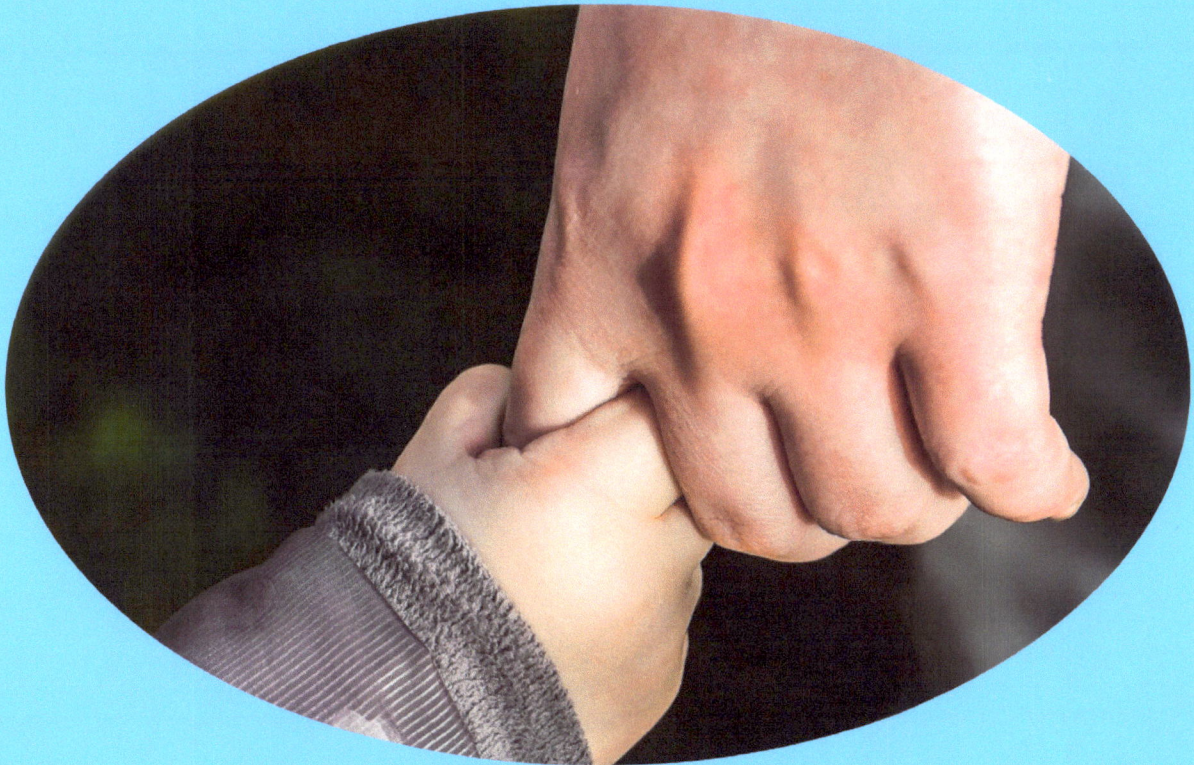

An Easy to Read Handbook for Children on Prevention and Awareness of Child Sexual Abuse with the supervision of Caregivers, Educators or Therapists.

"My Body Is Mine, Not Yours!"

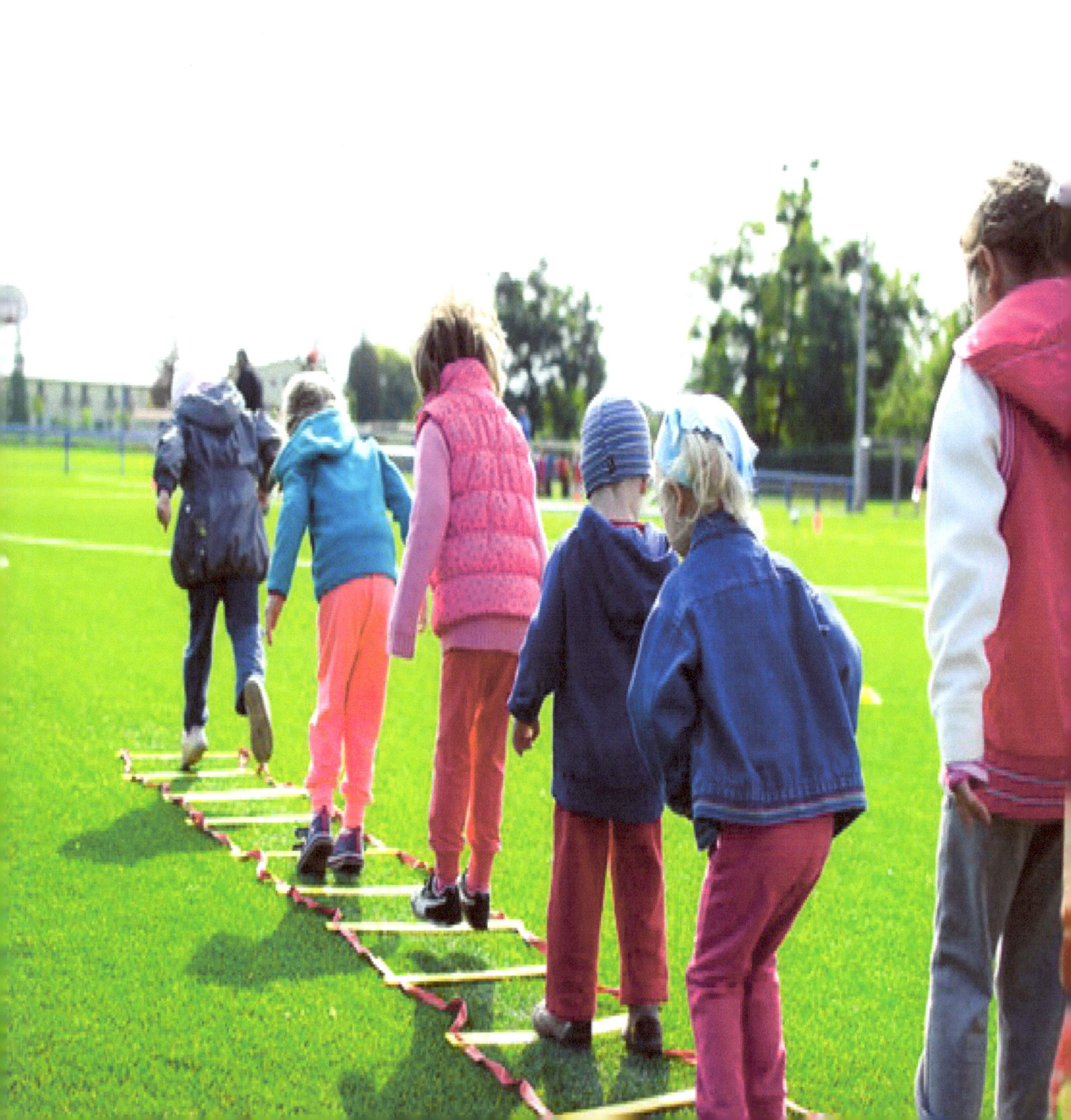

"My Body Is Mine, Not Yours!"

This is a book to help you understand about your body and how to look after it.

You will learn how special your body is and how to love, care and respect your body. Why? Because your body belongs to "only" you.

Let's learn about what are your personal private places. Look at the picture on the next page. It will give you an idea of the personal/private places on your body where you don't want people to touch.

The BLUE is your personal bubble. You have control over this space.

The RED is your private area. You have control over this space.

The YELLOW is your brain area where they might try to tell you things that are wrong "lies" or bad things. Even your brain needs protecting.

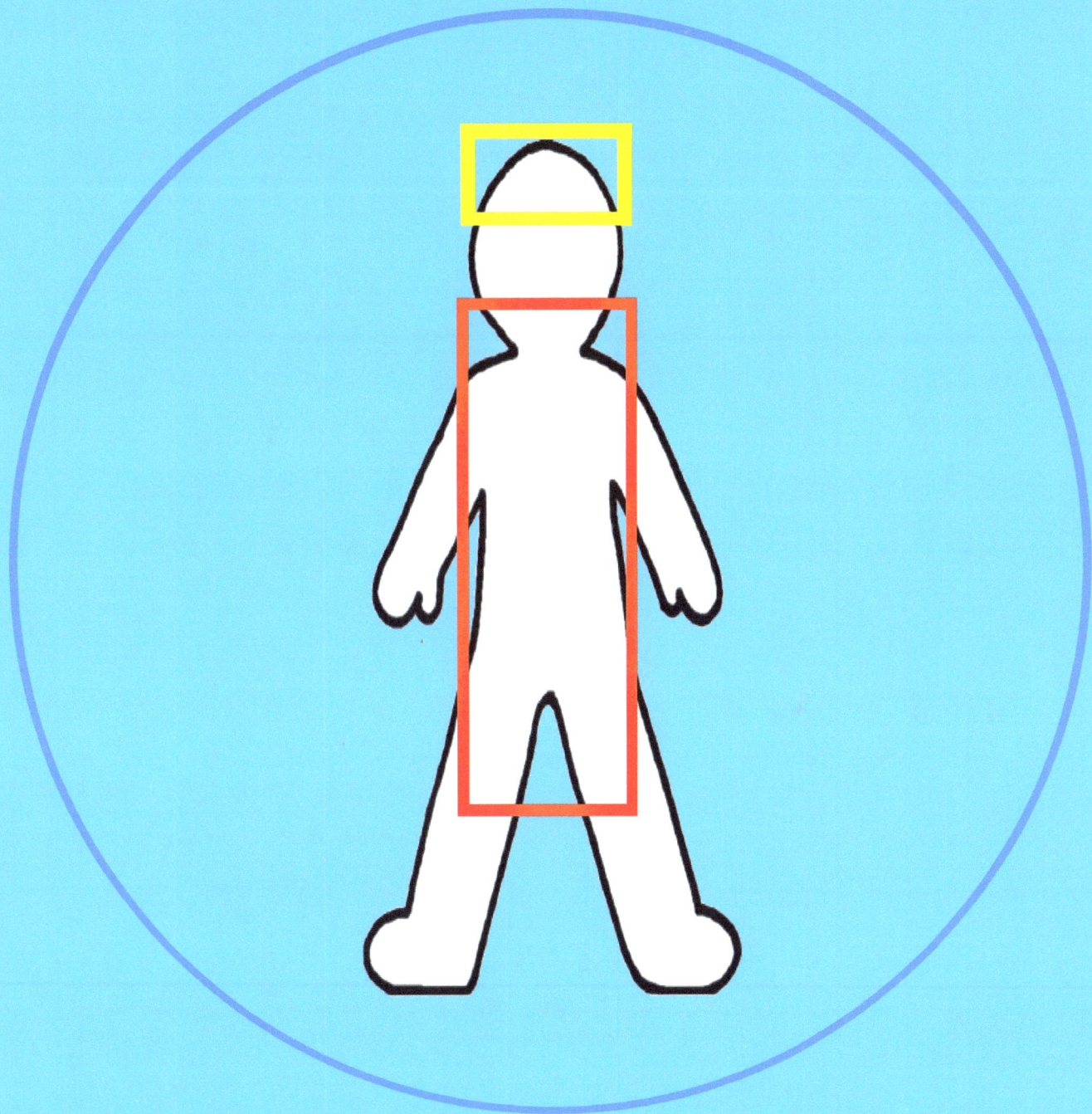

No one has the right to touch our private places except a doctor, parent or carer who may need to do this if you are sick in that area. But if you have a sore eye or ear or arm and your doctor, parent or carer touches you there then this is fine.

Sometimes though they "may" have to touch you in your private place "if" you are sick there.

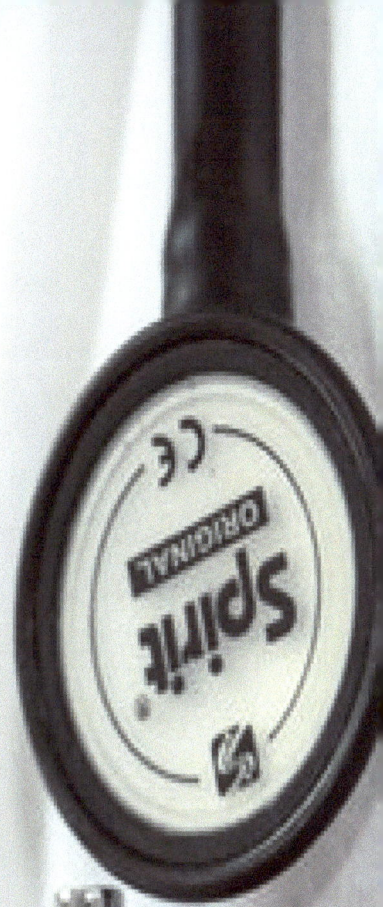

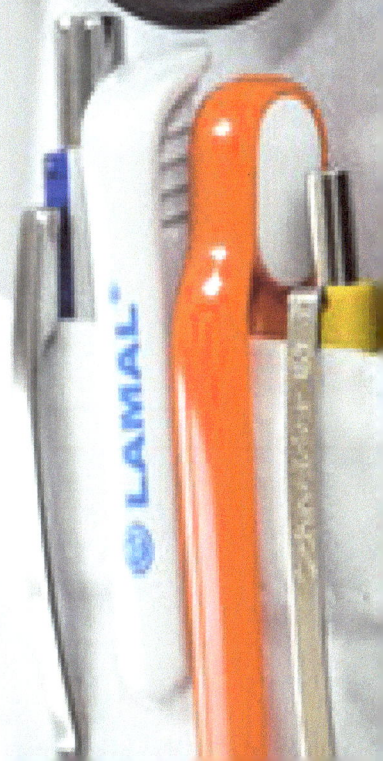

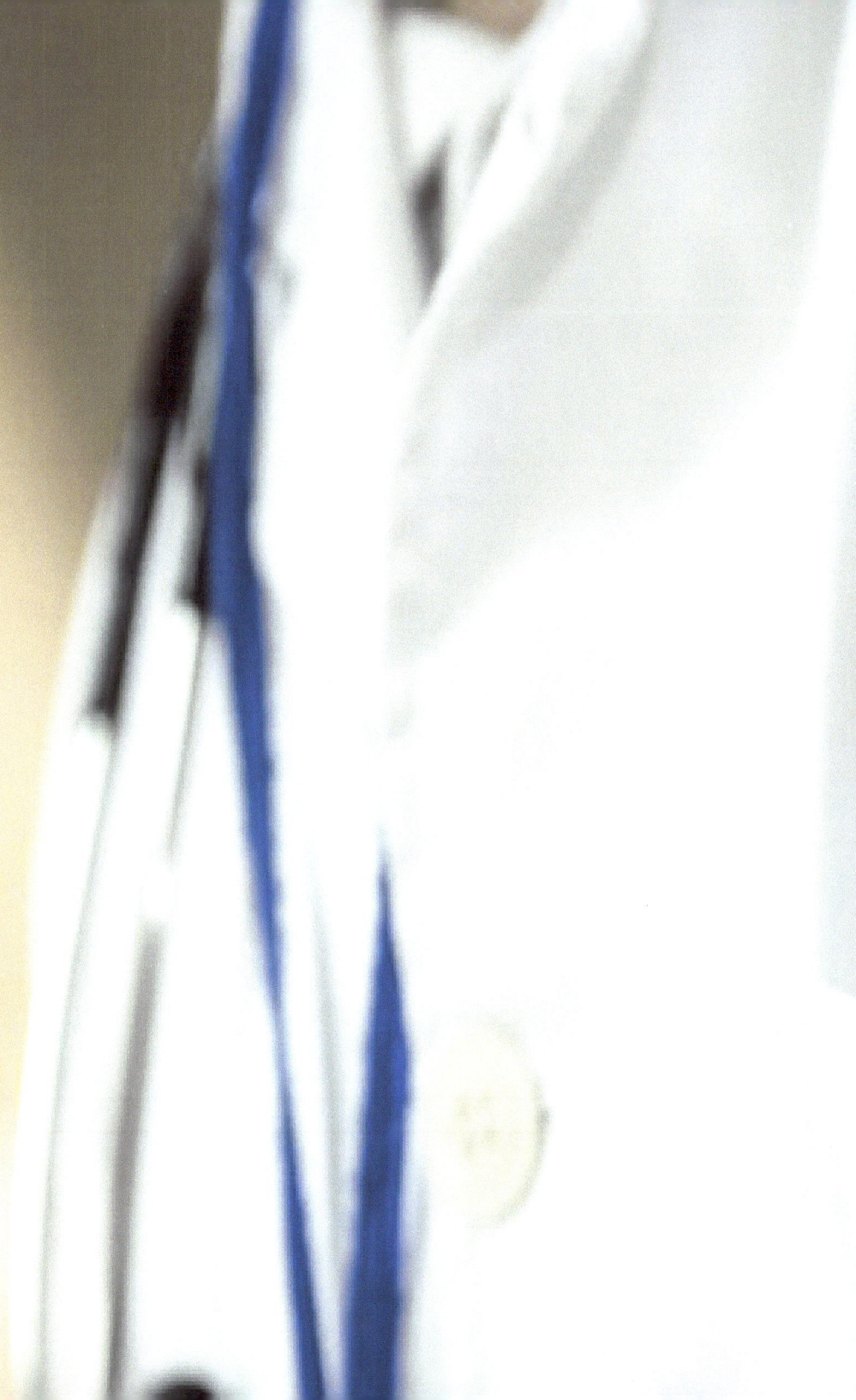

This is your body. Your body belongs to you, no one else.

If you are uncomfortable or nervous with the doctor you can ask for your parent, caregiver, or nurse to stay with you while the doctor looks at you.

Our bodies are called our personal space, sometimes it might feel uncomfortable if someone comes too close to us, this is ok, and it is a normal feeling. You "can" move away.

If you are uncomfortable you "should" let a trusted adult know. Why? Because it is right to feel safe and comfortable.

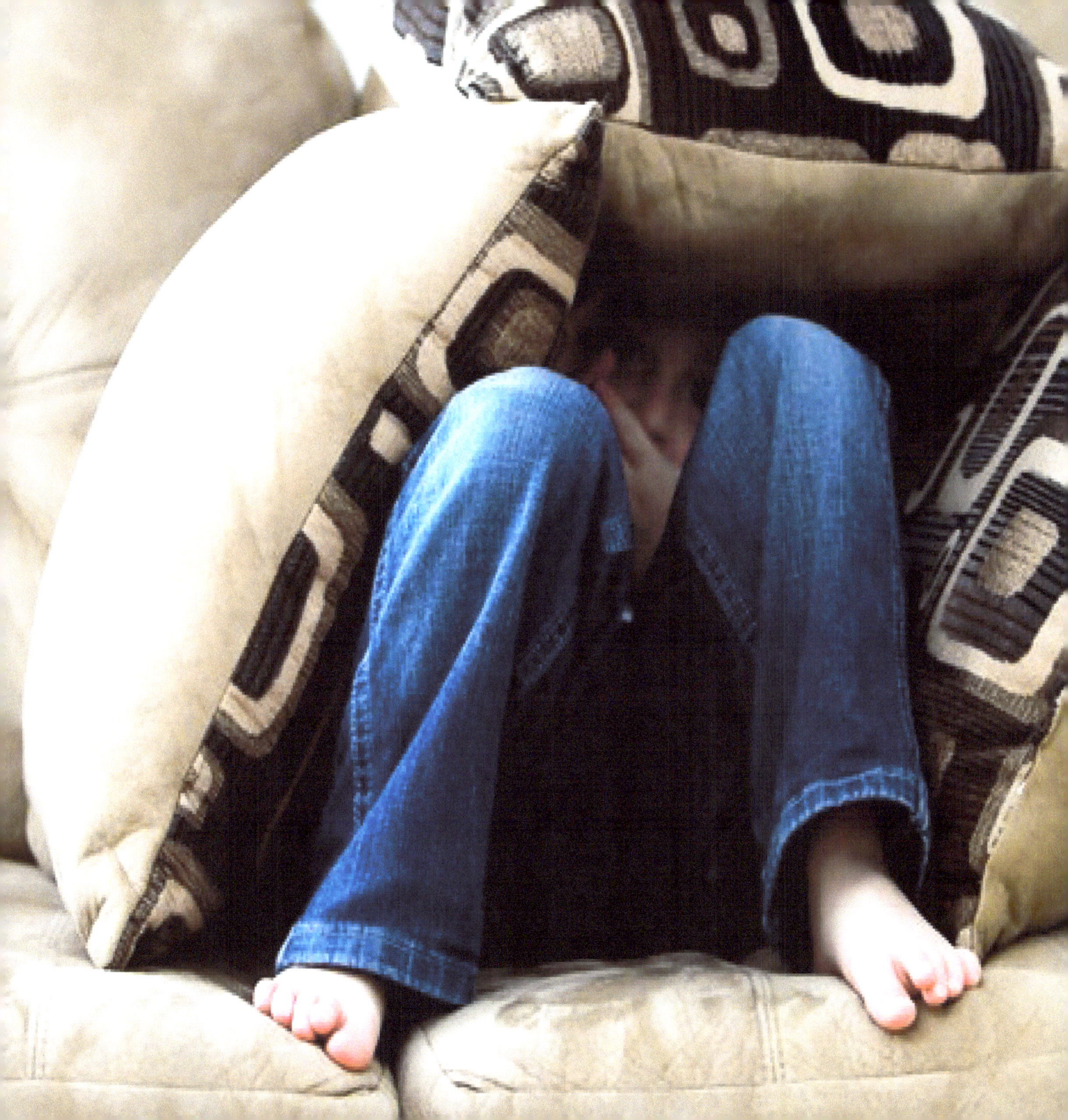

Stealing is when someone touches or takes something that does not belong to them.

Your body belongs to "only" you and it is good to protect what is yours.

Someone may touch you or ask you to touch their private place- "your" body, *It is wrong for them to do that to you.* ✗

Some people touch things that don't belong to them, this is wrong, this is called stealing.

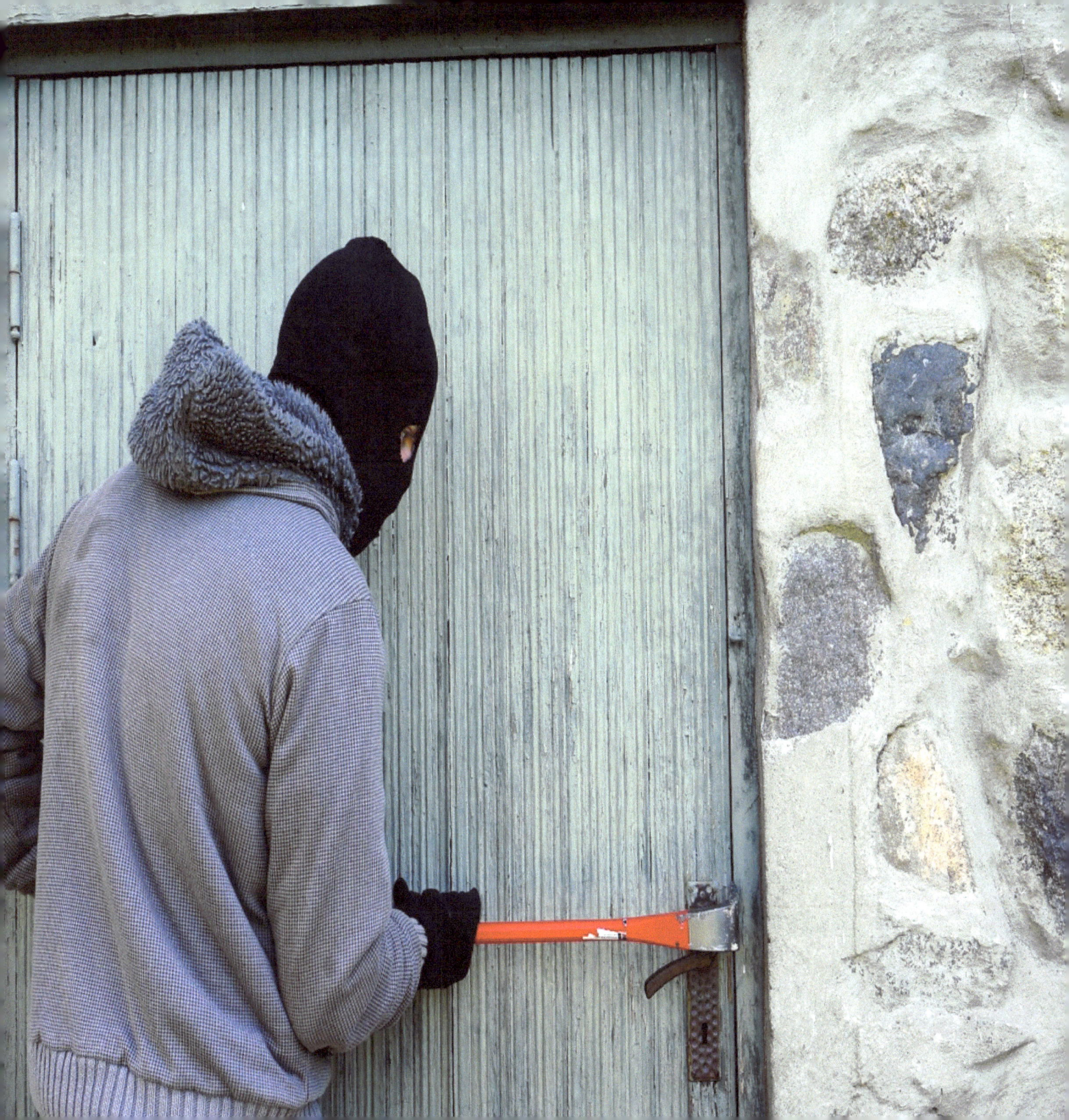

When our bodies are still growing it is hard to make our bodies stop feeling things.

It is wrong for this person to touch you in your private places, even though they may say that they are making you feel good.

Sometimes when they touch you it can feel good, don't feel bad it's not your fault. This is a normal feeling.

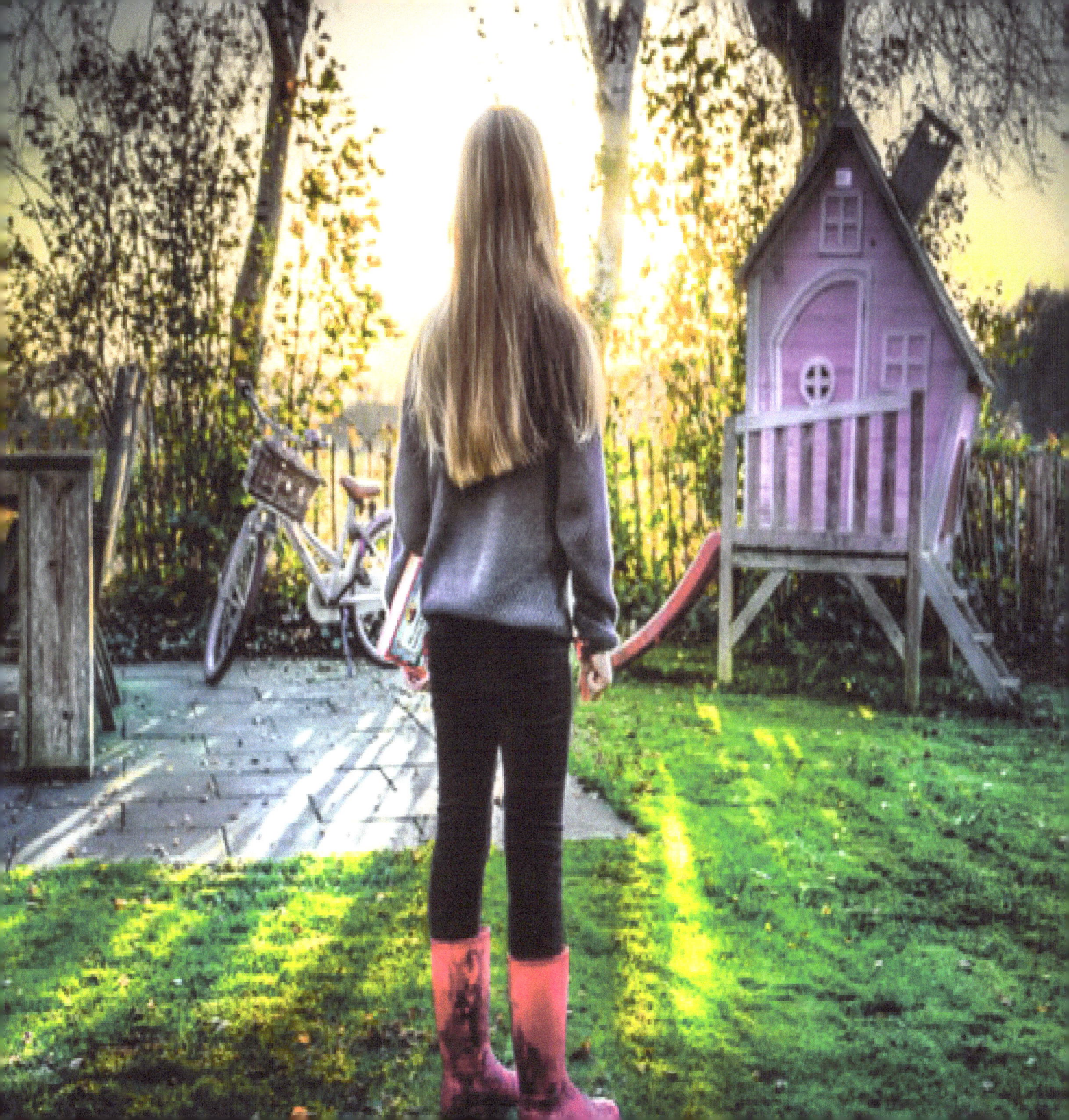

If that person makes you touch them in their private place or show you their private place, this is wrong too.

Remember "they" are in the wrong for making you do this, "not" you. This is "not" your fault.

Big people (Grown-ups/Adults) know better and should not do the wrong thing by you.

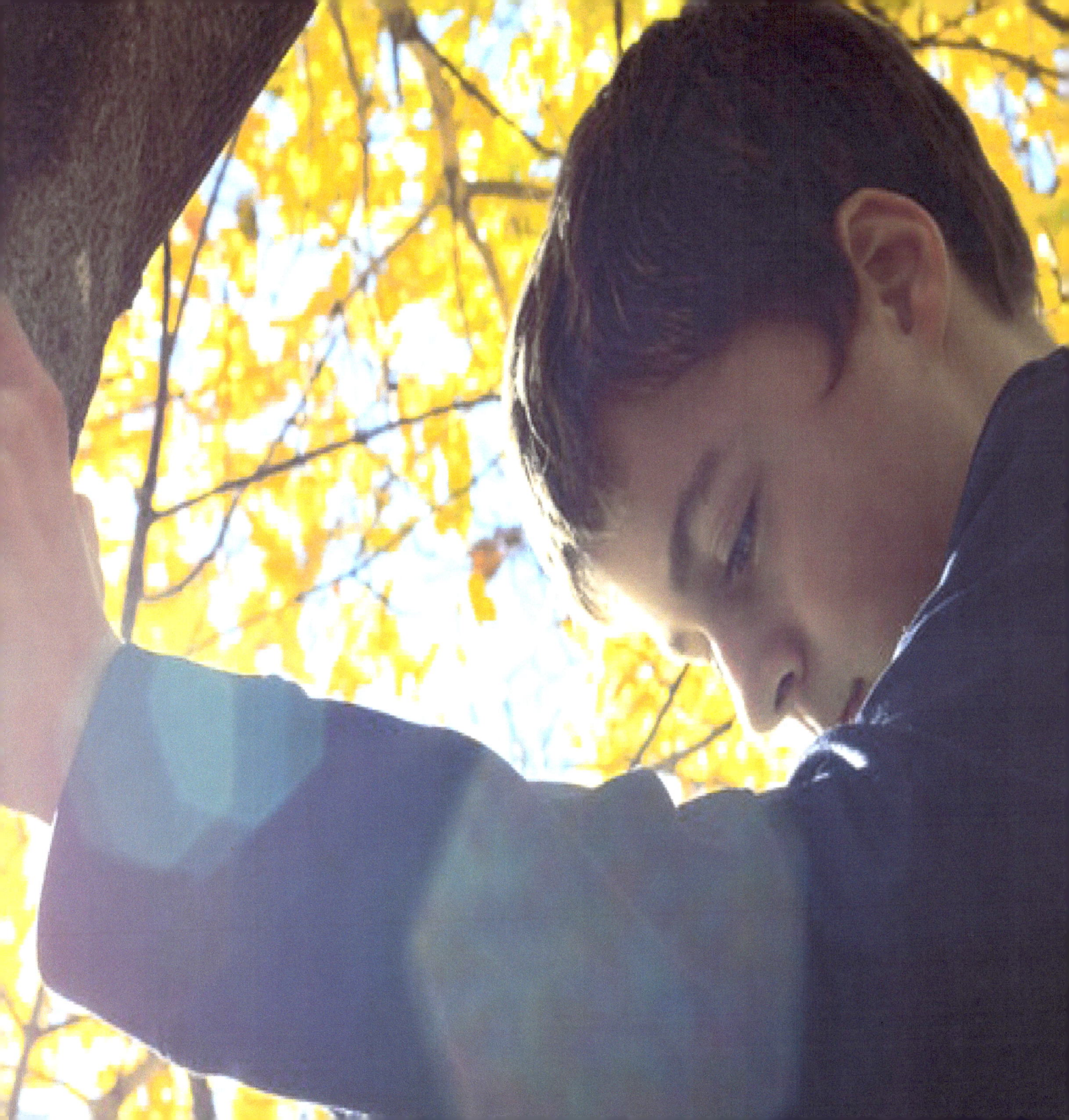

If someone touches you in your private places or makes you touch them or look at them you should say "NO!" and go and find another adult, a bigger person you can trust to tell.

This person can be your Aunt, your Dad or a Teacher, someone like that.

Just make sure it is someone you feel safe to talk to, that you know will listen.

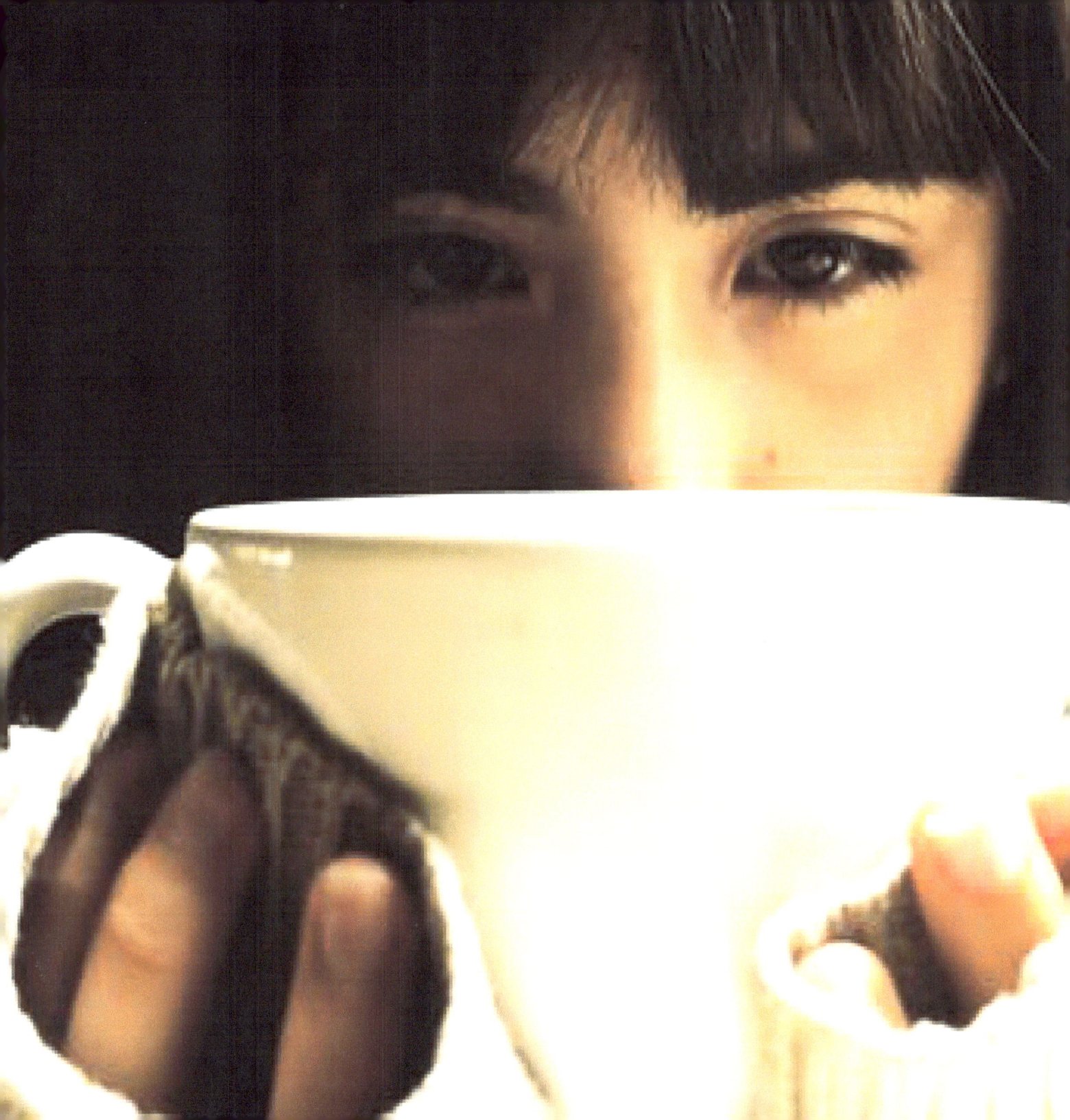

It is ok and good for you to stand up for yourself and tell a trusted adult and say "NO!"✓

Some big people do wrong things; just because they are bigger than you it does not mean no one else will believe you.

You should "always" tell someone, an adult you trust if this has happened to you.

Don't worry that someone might not believe you, because someone will "always" believe you.

If someone touched, you in your private place or made you touch them. Remember you did "nothing" wrong.

It was the person that touched you or made you touch them that did something wrong, "not" you.

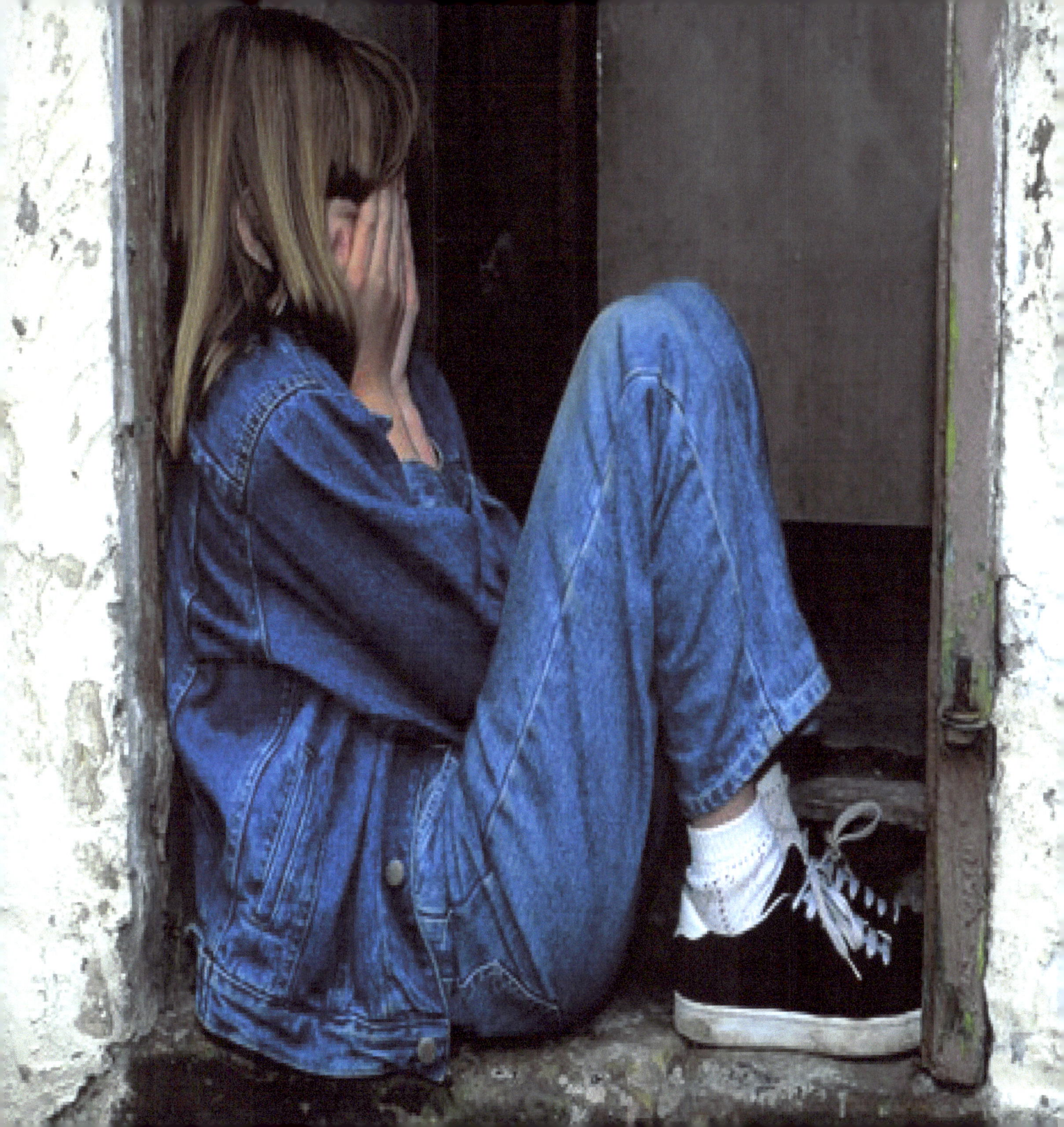

It could be your Uncle, Aunt, Grandpa, Grandma, your Friend, Mum, Dad, Step Parent, Teacher, Doctor or even someone from kids' camp; it could be anyone you know that has touched you in the wrong place. It is very "sad", but it can sometimes happen.

Most people are not like this. Even though people sometimes do things that are wrong doesn't make them a bad person, it is just that they really need help. It can all be so hard to understand. You "will" feel better when you talk about your feelings to a caring person.

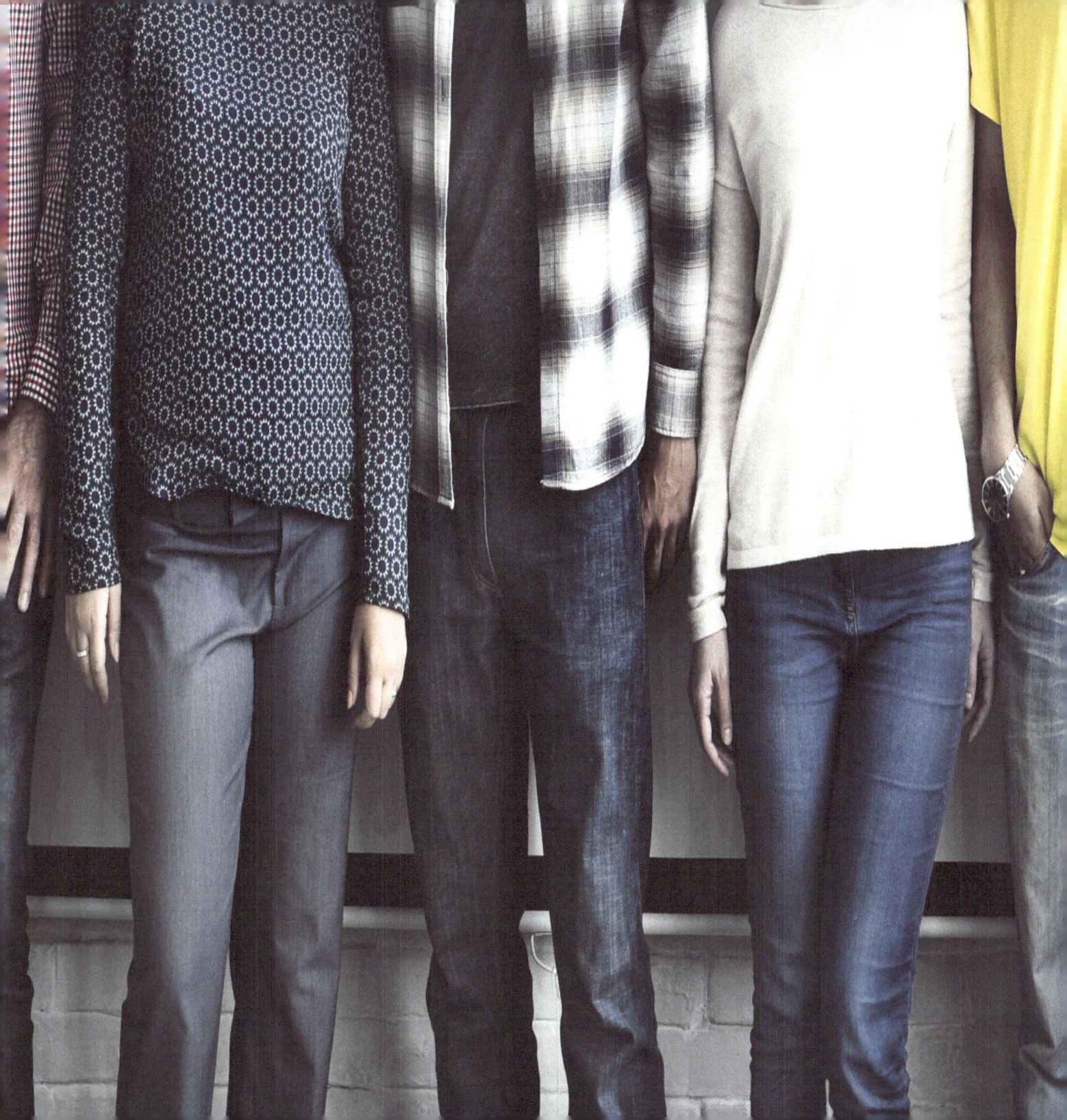

Tell a caring grown up who you think will listen. Someone might want to take "photos" of you with your personal/private place, this is wrong too. You can say, "No don't!" or Don't touch me!" ✓

If this happens you need to tell your mum, dad, teacher or someone older that you can trust. This is not called dobbing; it is called looking after yourself.

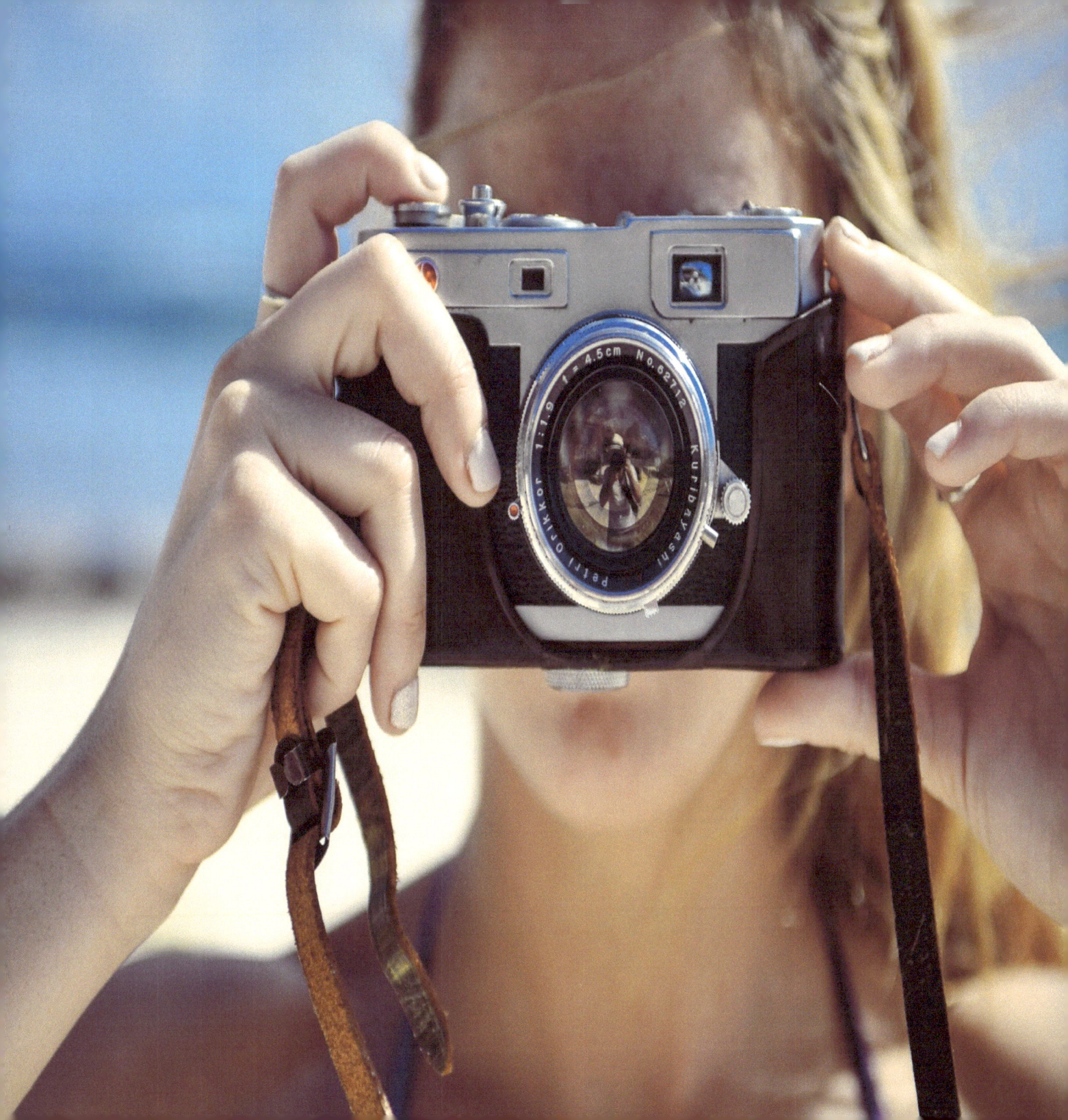

If someone goes to touch you in your private/personal places or gives you certain kisses or hugs that don't feel right, you can speak up and say, **"Please don't hug me."** or **"Please don't kiss me, I don't like it."**✓

You "can" say this even if they are family.

It is "not" being rude.

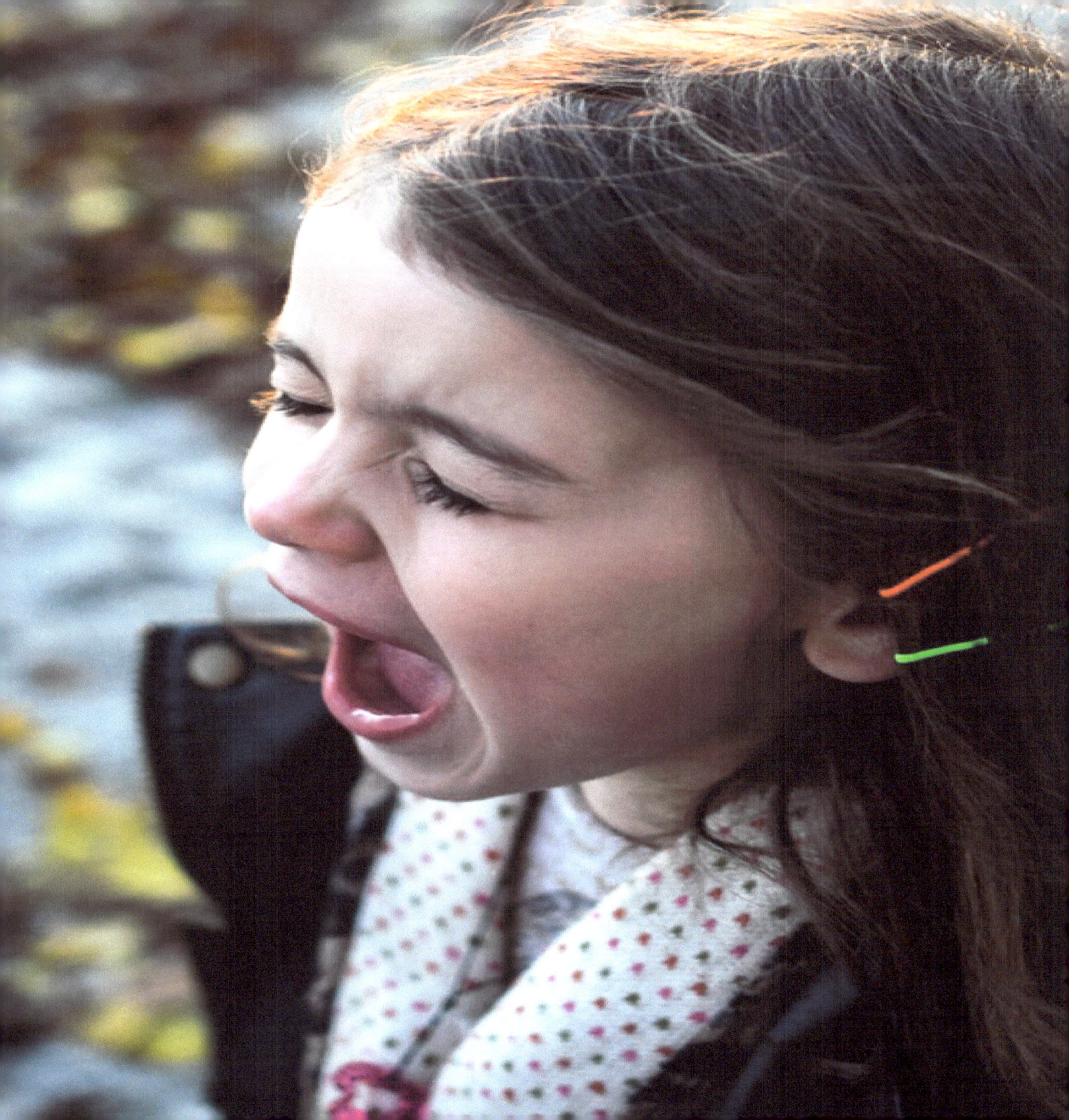

If someone wants you to stay over their house for the night and you don't want to. You have the right to say, "No thank you." √

You can also tell a trusted adult if you don't want to do certain things.

This could also be a good time to let your Mum, Dad or someone you trust know about your feelings or if anything has been happening to you.

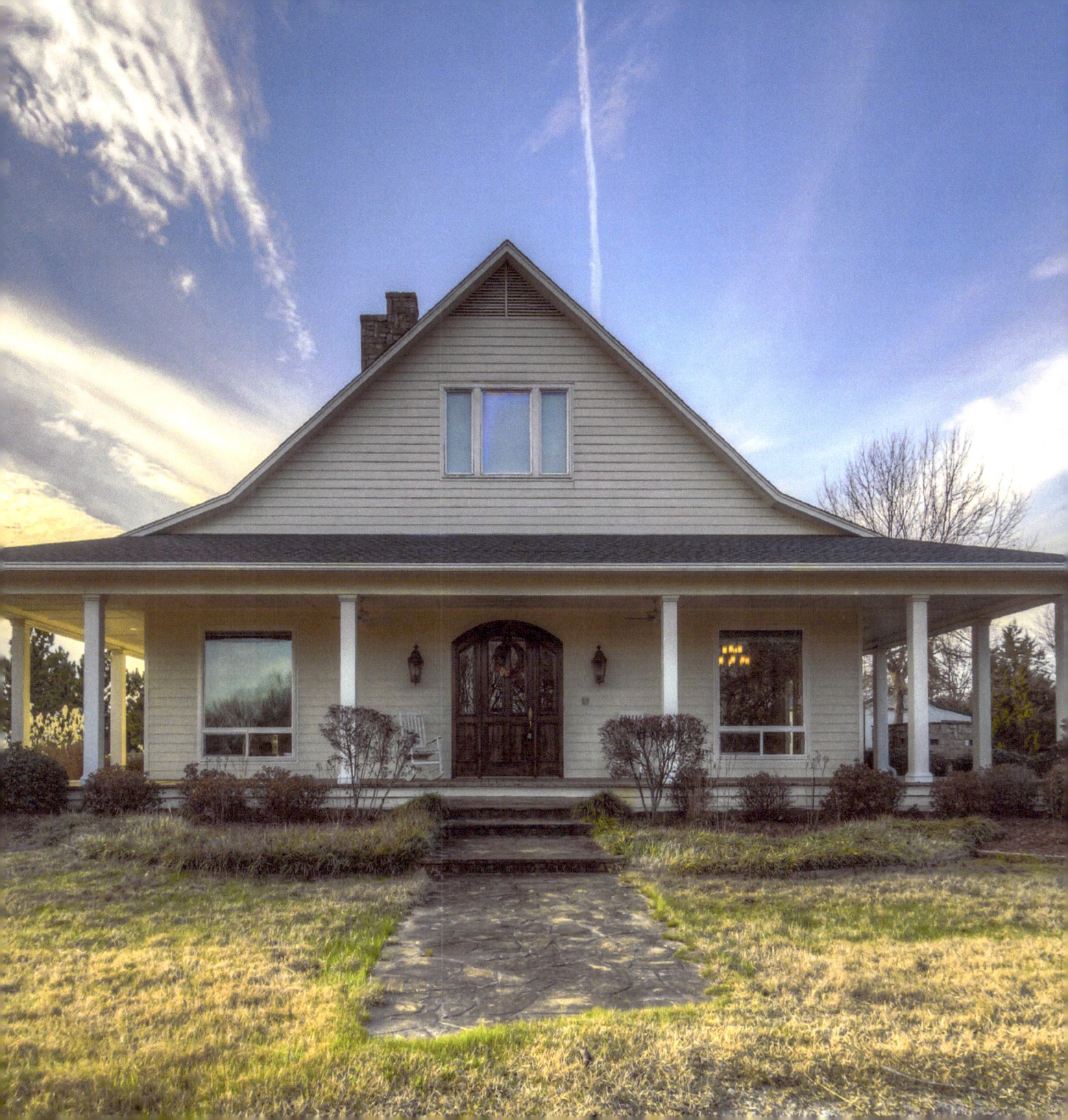

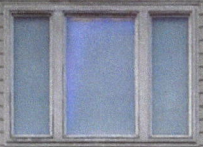

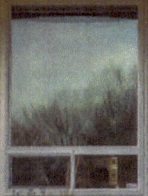

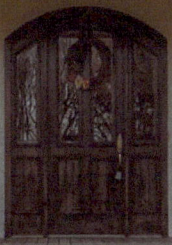

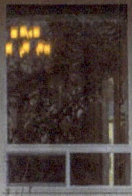

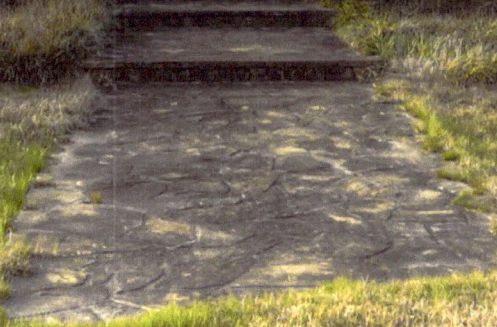

Someone may want to take you in their car or say, "Come with me so you can pat my puppy," × or they may try to give you candy, ice-cream, toys or money. Be careful they could be trying to trick you and take you away. They might have a cute puppy.

But do you really need to pat it? No, you can pat puppies when you are with someone you trust.

Do "not" go with them. Some people pretend to be good people.

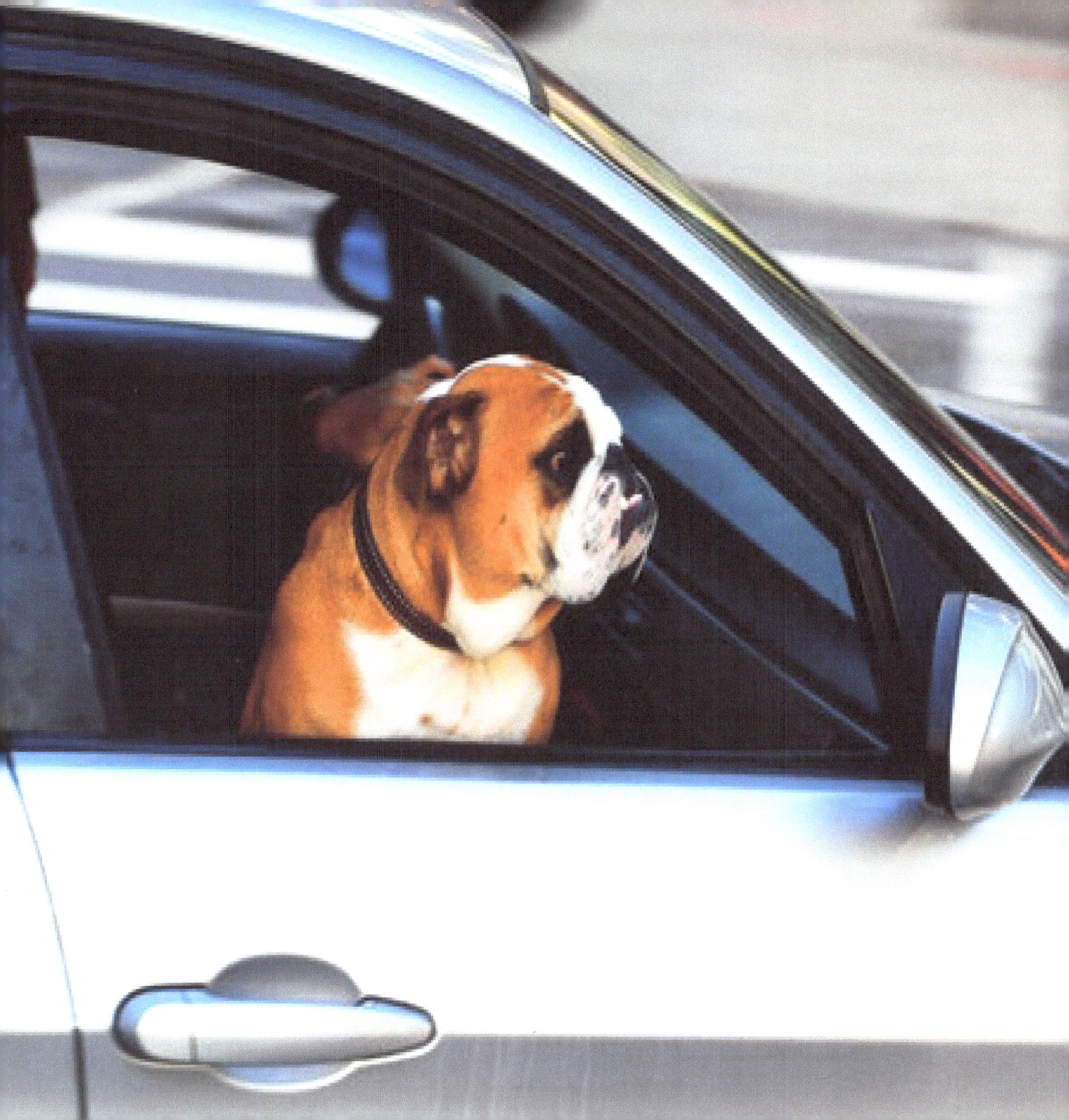

Do you know this person or people?

How well do you know them?

Do "not" go with them.

Do they know the secret password your Mum or Dad gave you?

"Can you trust them?"

You don't really know.

The person could be lying and trying to trick you.

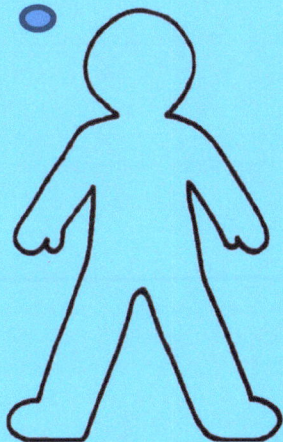

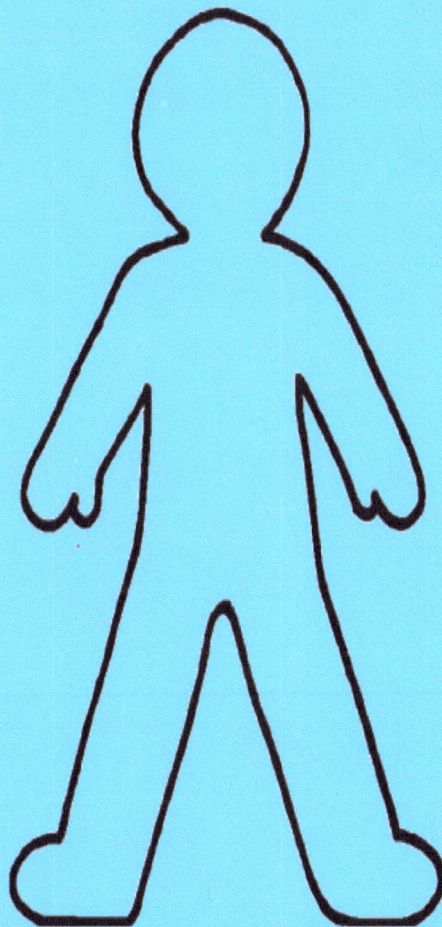

Using computers and mobile/cell phones can be fun and interesting. We still need to be careful when we use these items.

When you are talking on computer or phone, think to yourself, "Is this person ok?"

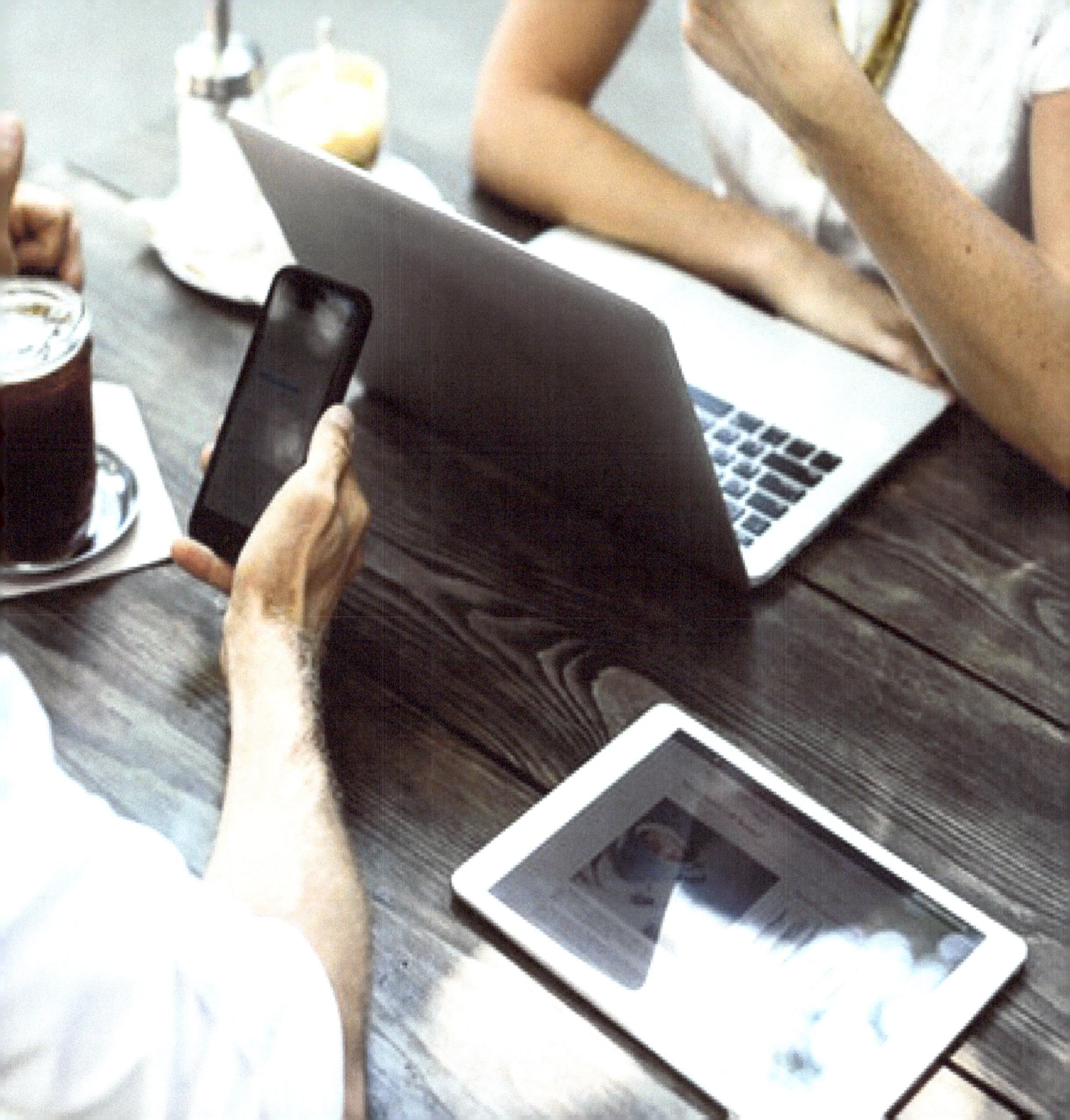

The park is a great place to go for fun. But still be careful.

If a person says, *"Meet me at the shops or at the park."* ×

Do "not" go.

"Never" tell them where you live and do "not" give them your phone number or address that is private. You don't even have to tell them your name if you don't want to.

Tell an adult you think you can trust straight away.

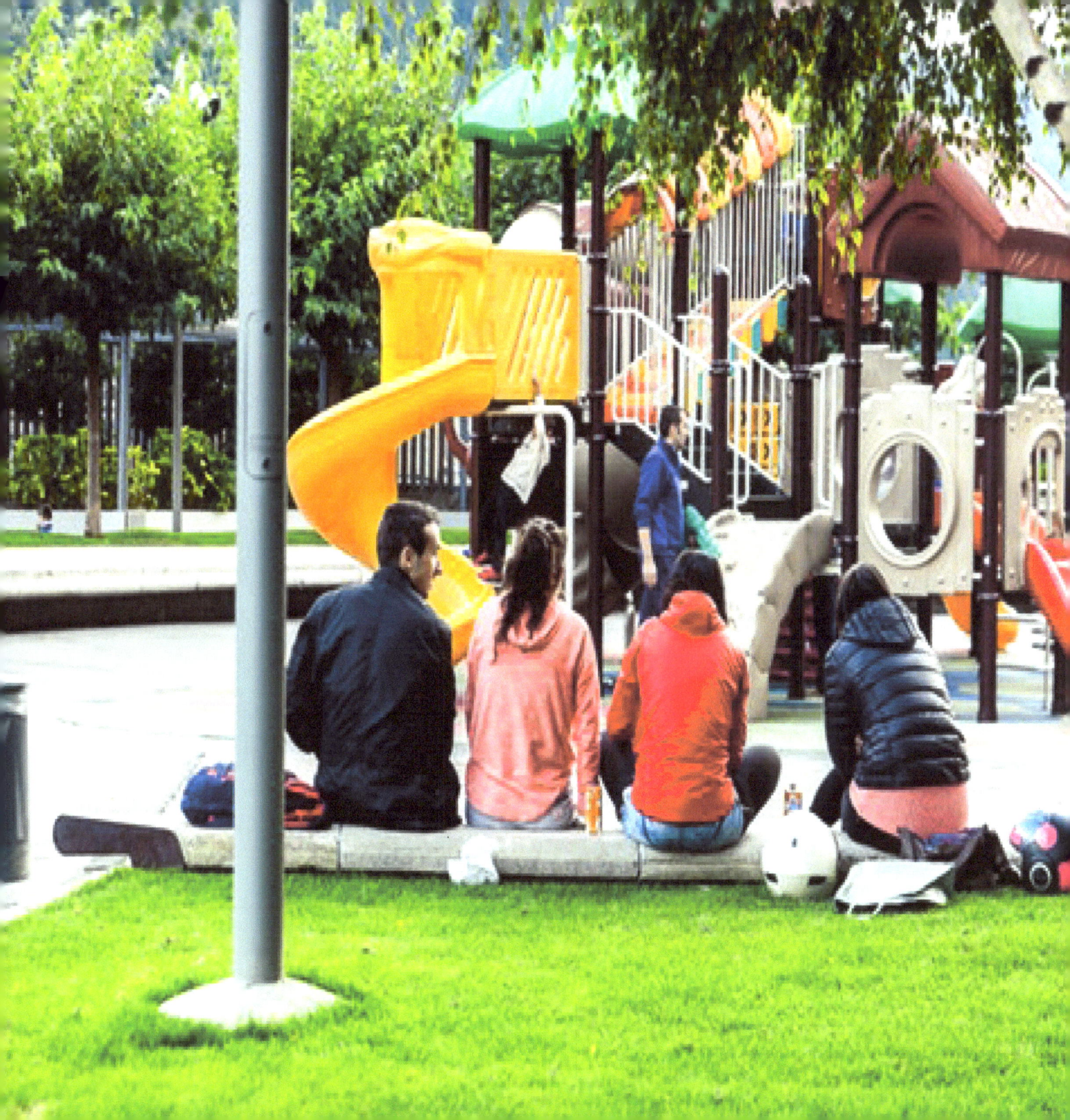

Someone may say don't tell anyone or they may say to you, *"It's our secret."*× This is when it is "not" good to keep a secret.

Sometimes the person who did the wrong thing may be mean and say, "This is a secret and if you tell I will hurt your mum, dad, someone else or you."× You must still tell.√

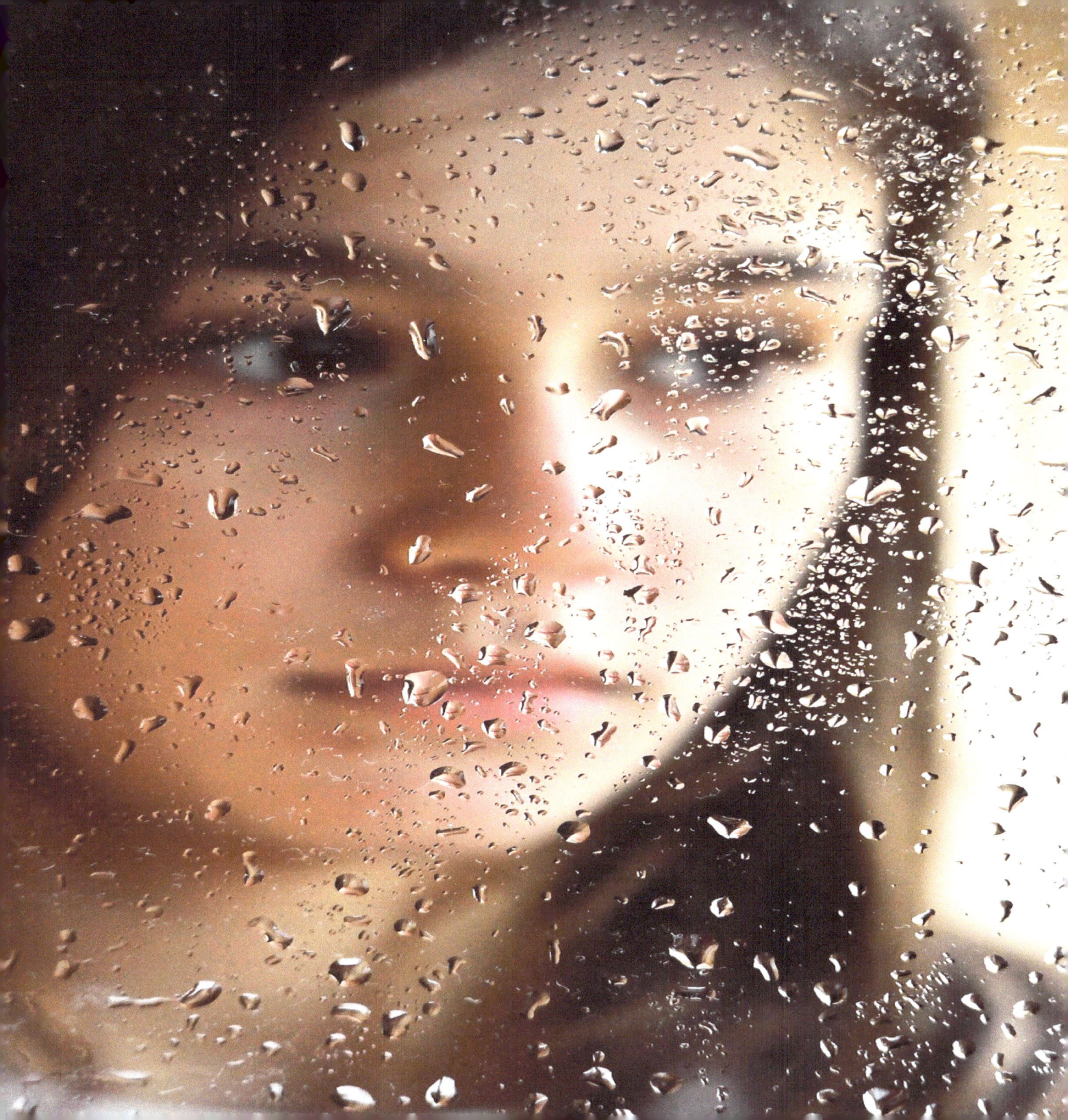

You need to tell a caring grown up, your mum, dad, a teacher, a relative.

'Don't' let them bully you. You "can" be brave! √

Bullies can be adults or children; people you know or don't know.

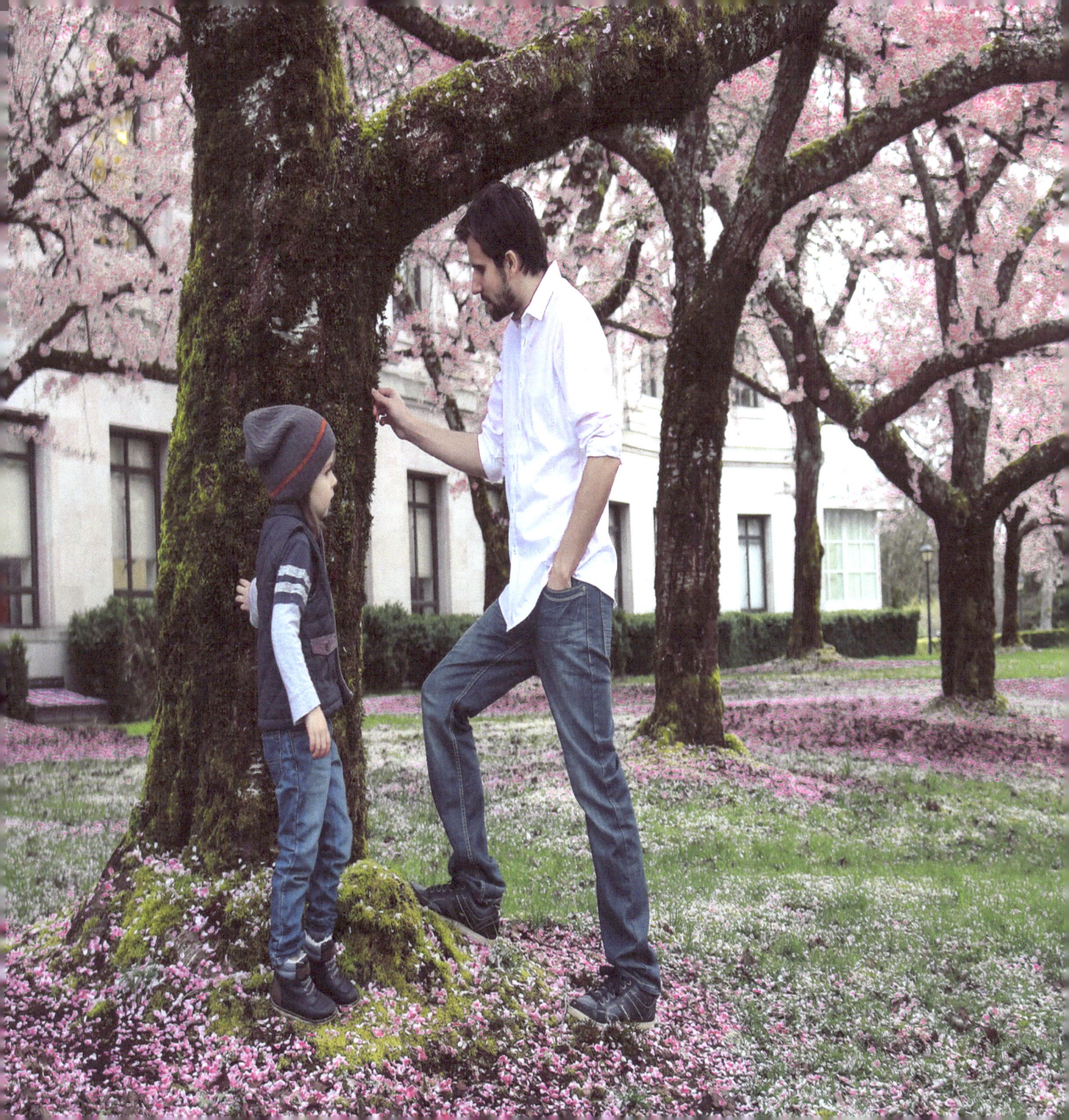

When we are sad it is good to talk, to be able to talk about our feelings to Mum or Dad or someone like your Teacher or close friend.

Sometimes we think no one will understand or care. There is "always" someone who will understand and does care about you.

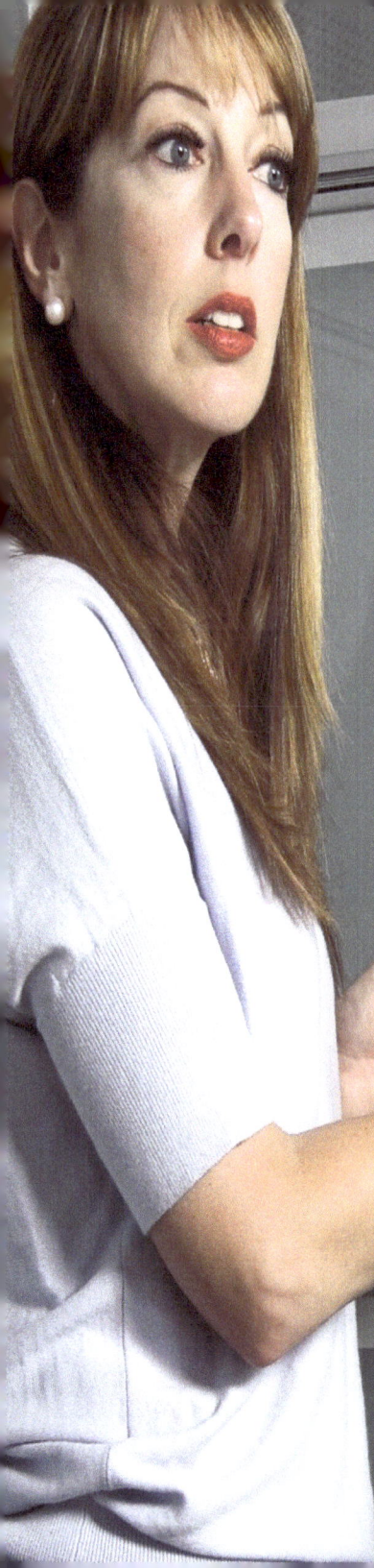

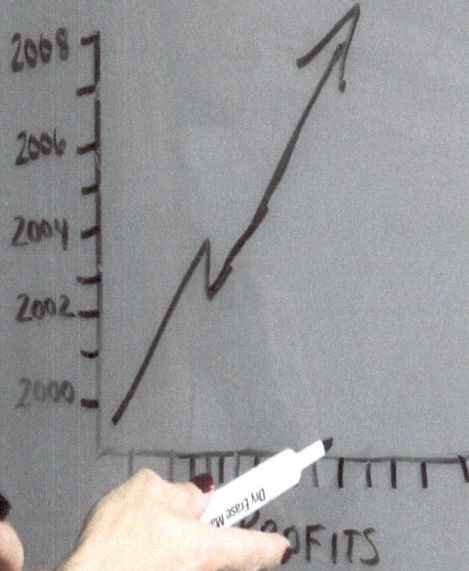

The person you trusted to tell will do all they can to protect look after you or your loved ones. So, do not worry about telling. Telling is "good" and it is the "right" thing to do. You won't get into trouble.

Remember "no one" can help you if you don't speak up and tell. Because they won't know you need help.

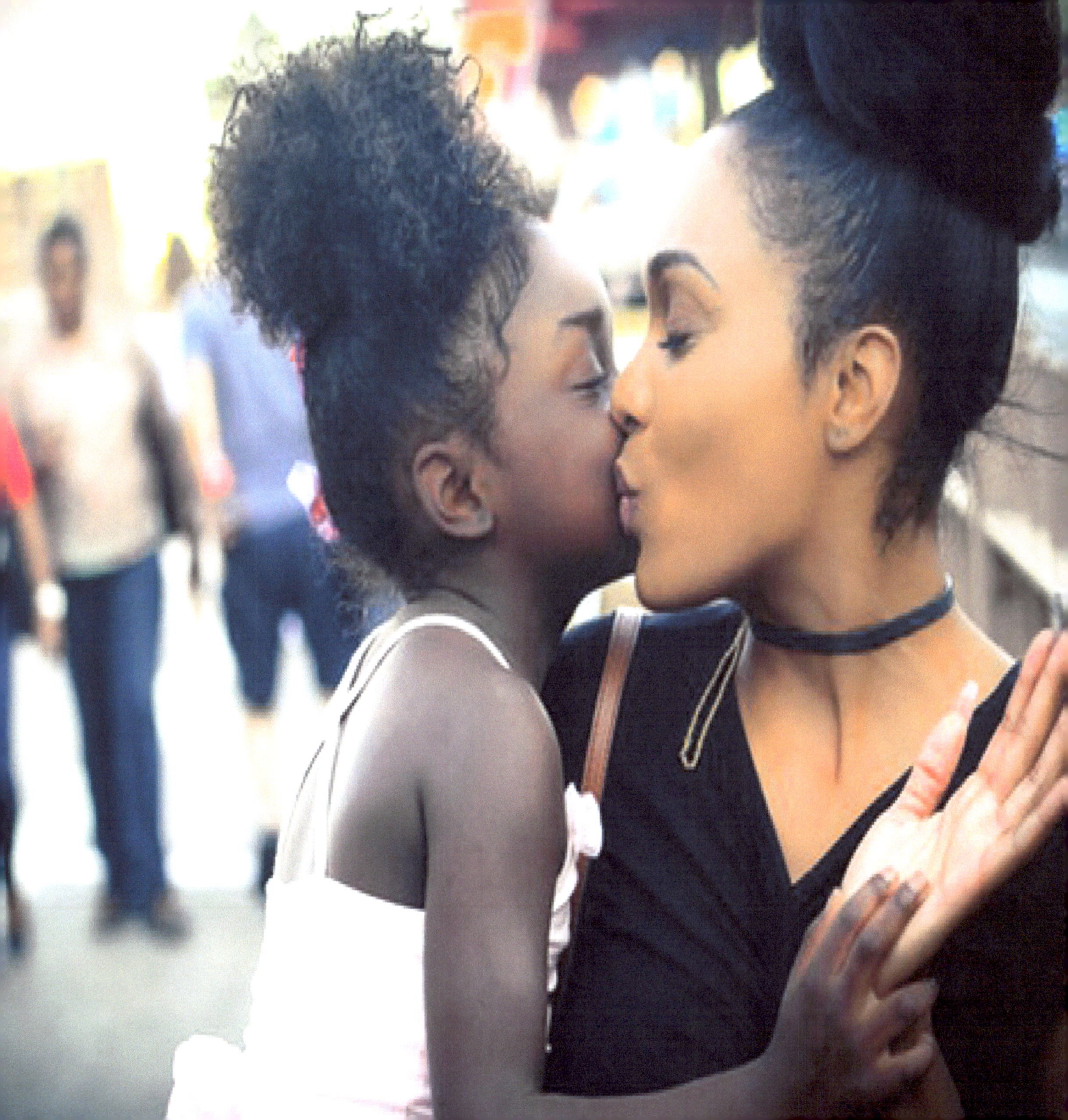

So, to help yourself "you need to tell someone who you think will listen to you." Please try not to be afraid.

If you know of this happening to you, your brother or sister, your friend or someone else? You "can" get them some help by telling an adult that you trust will help. This is a good thing you are doing.√

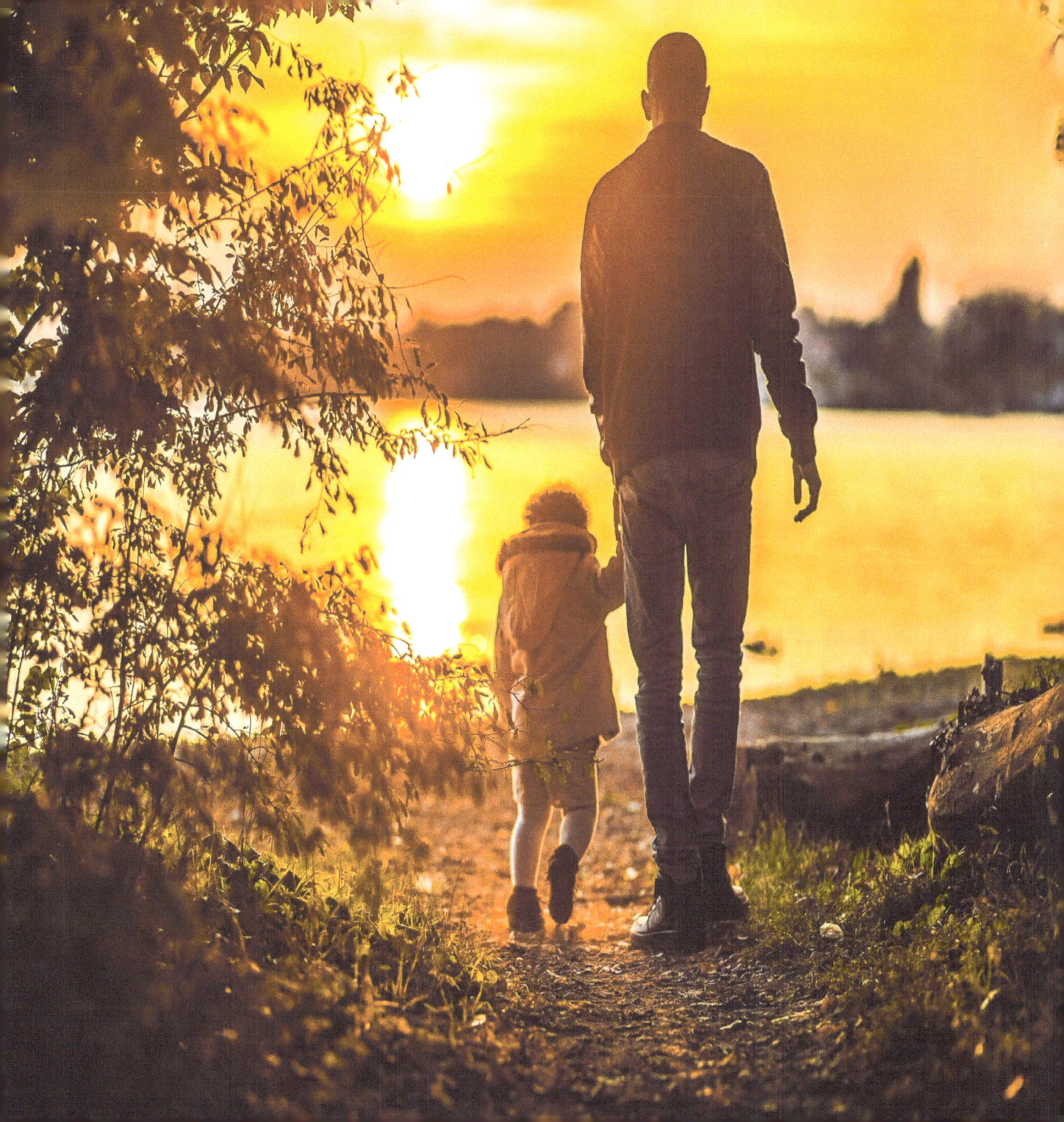

Remember, again a trusting adult could be; your Teacher, Mum or Dad. Be brave and tell someone you can trust. Even if it is about someone you know.

You "must" tell a trusted adult. This person could be the school nurse, your doctor, teacher or parents. Really you are helping the other person and yourself. They "can" go to a doctor for help. So really you are doing the right thing. It's "not" your fault. ✓

Try not to be scared, you are doing a good thing.

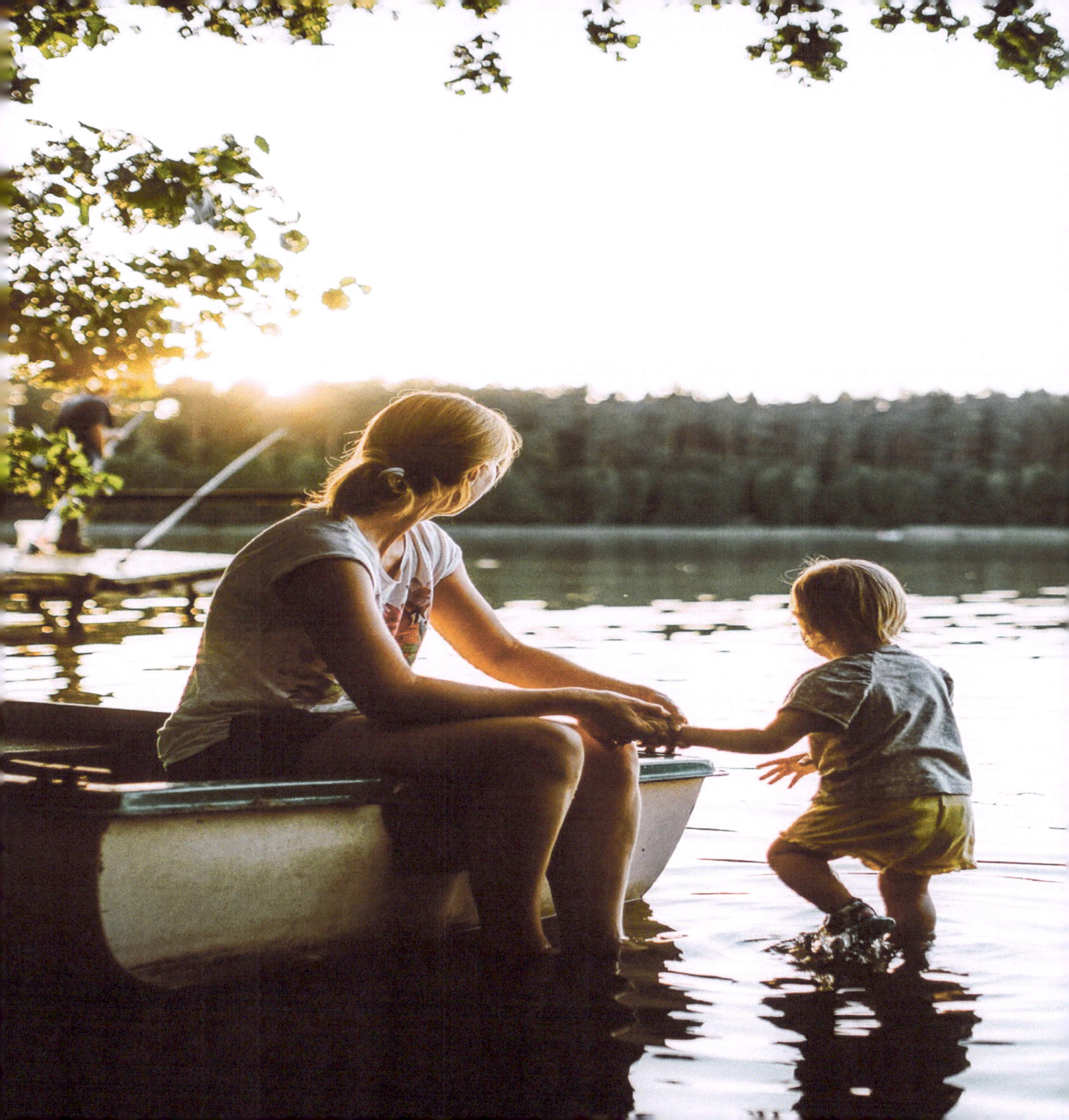

The person you trusted to tell, will do all they can to protect and help you. So now do not worry about telling. Telling is good, telling is the right thing to do. "You are a good person!"

Talking about our feelings is very important; it helps the other person understand us better. You will also feel better too. Being alone with your worries and feelings is "not" good for you.

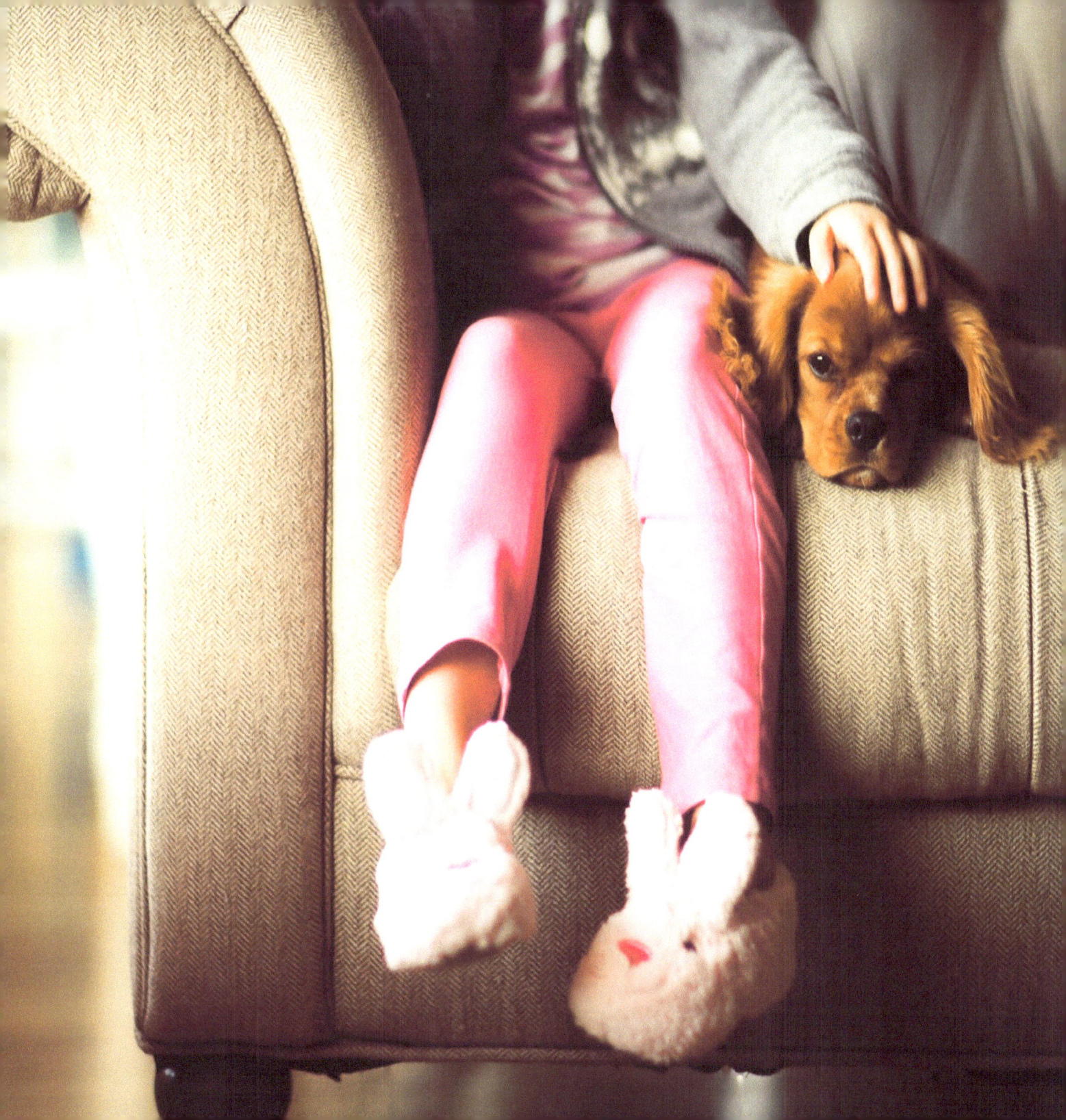

Something else that can be uncomfortable is tickling. You can nicely say "Stop!" "I don't like it!" √ Not many people like tickling, so it's normal not to like it. It's ok not to like it. You may notice that sometimes animals like it more than people.

Over time you will learn that there are other children that may have had this happen to them. You are not alone.

Maybe nothing will ever happen to you, which is good; but it is also good to know "how" to look after yourself.

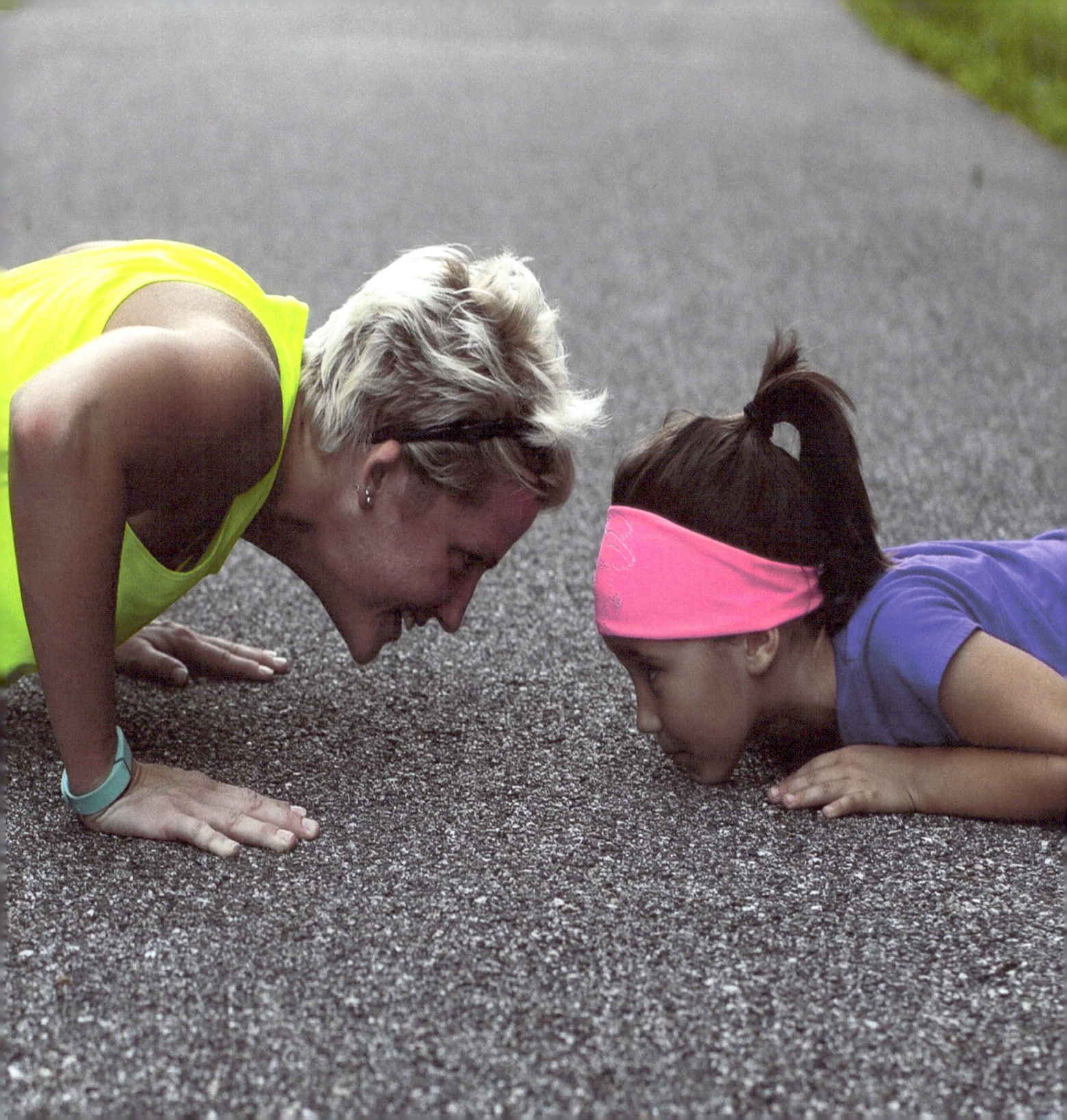

Always know that "you are important."

You "can" look after yourself. You "can" say "Leave me alone!" or "Don't touch me!"✓ You can even scream if you want to. Practise saying it with someone you trust.

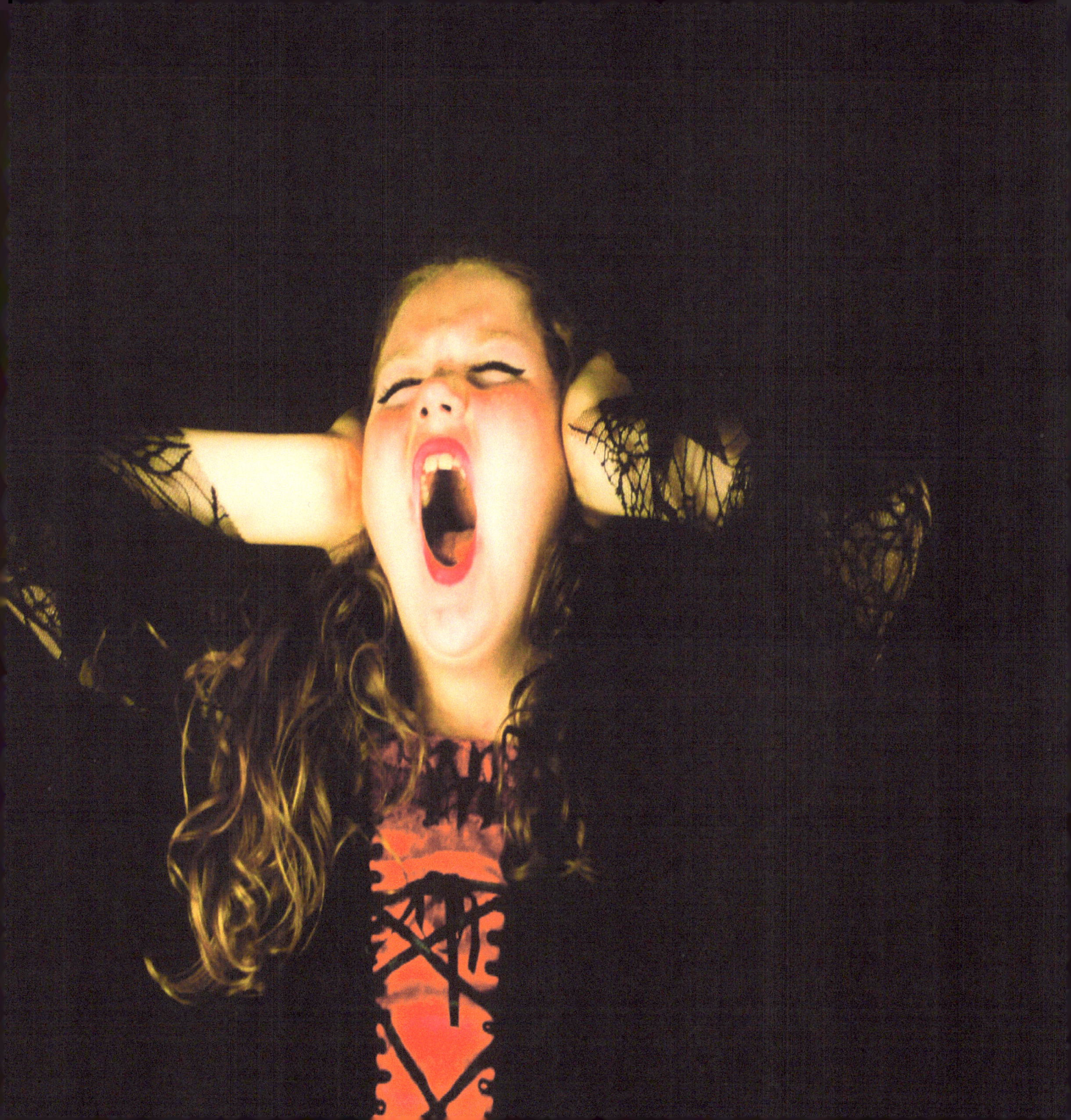

When you do tell someone you trust, never be scared, because someone will "always" listen and believe you.

Always remember "My Body Is Mine, Not Yours!" ✓

Remember your body is "yours" and no one really needs to touch it.

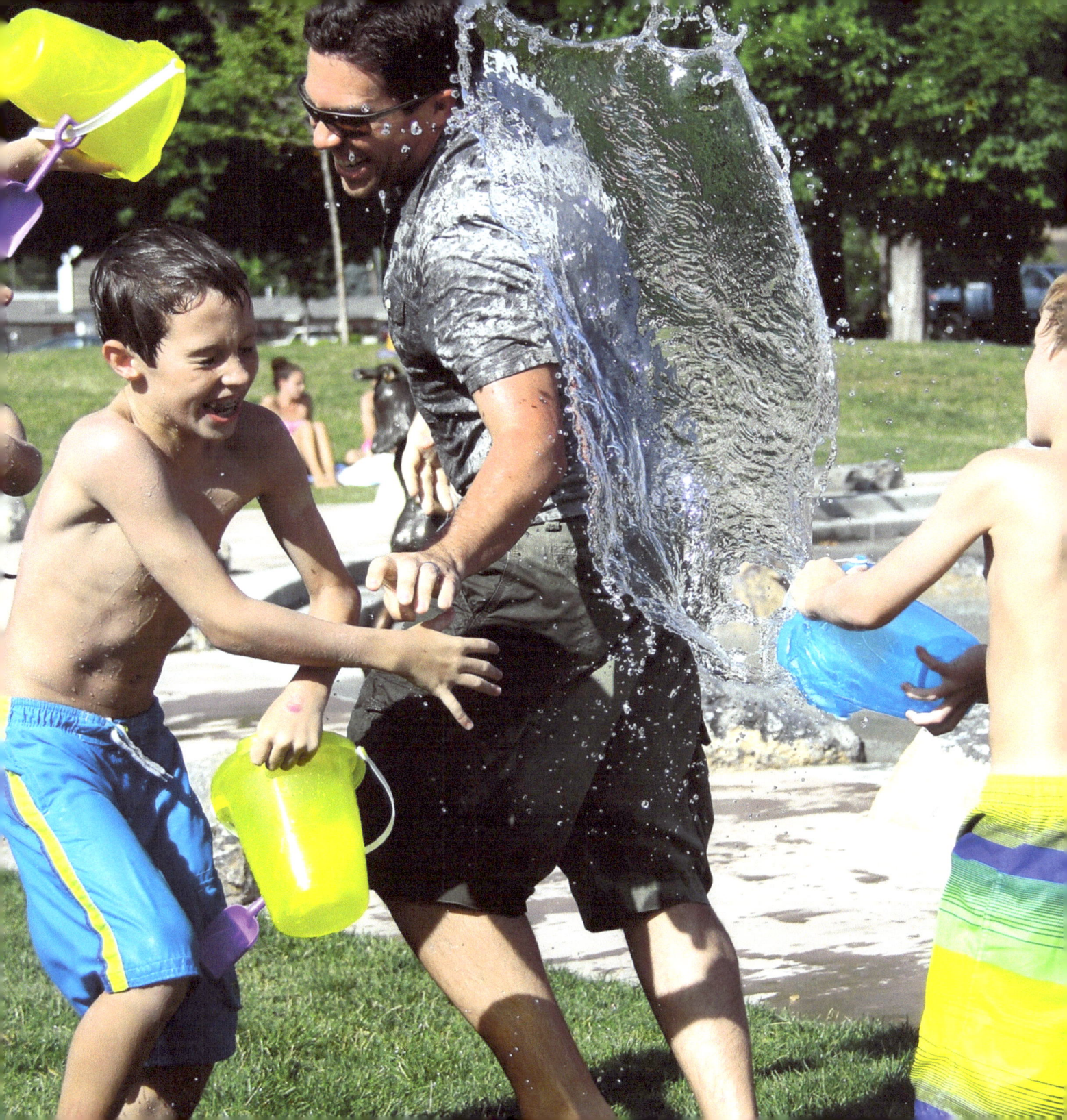

You "can" say to yourself;

I am a good person.
I am brave.
I am strong.
I can protect myself.
I can tell if I need to.

To end this lesson, let's remember that you are strong, and no matter what you will never be alone.

THE END

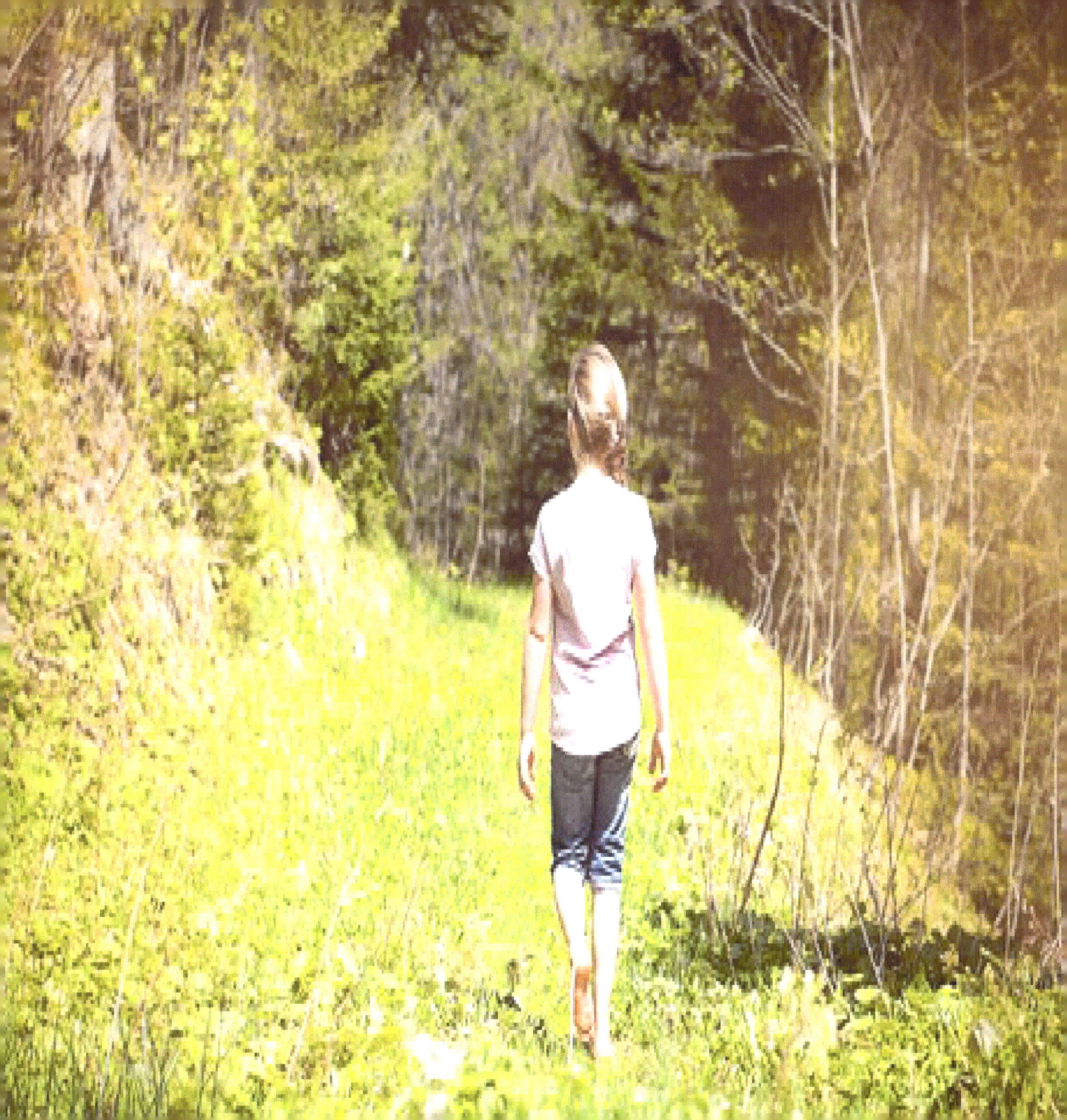

Remember Always;

"My Body Is Mine, Not Yours!"

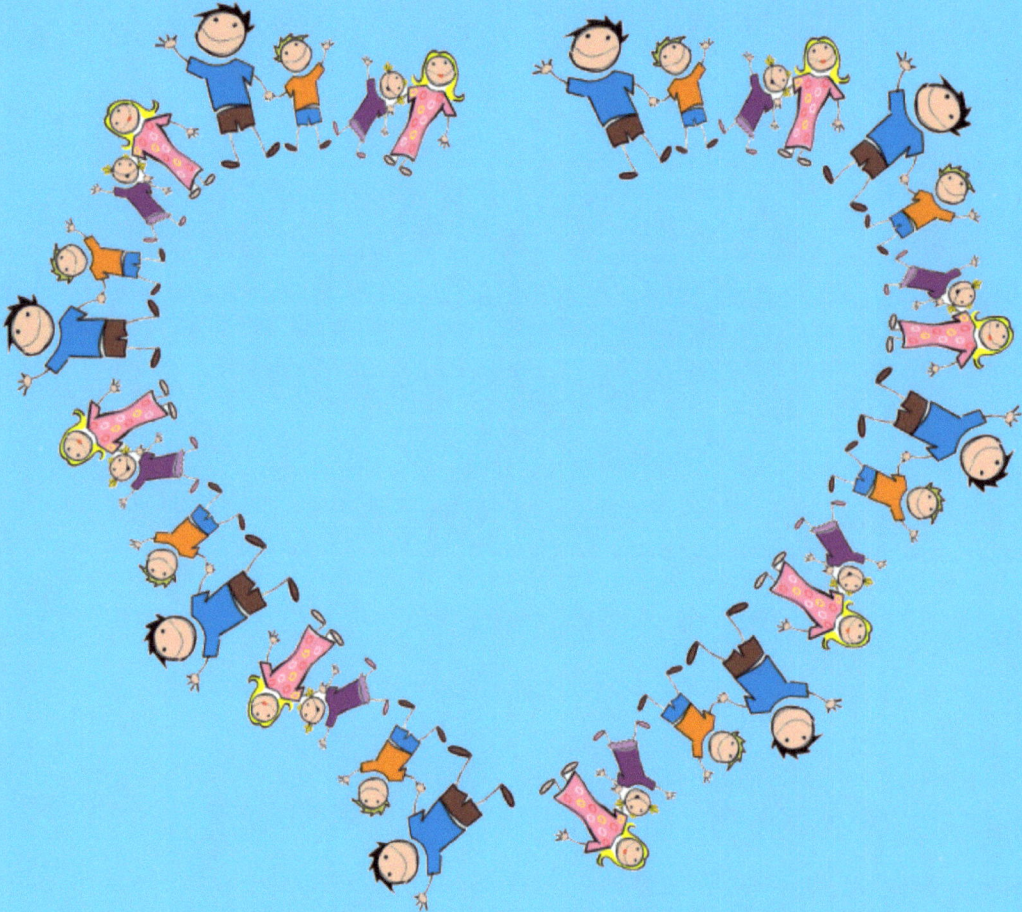

"My Body Is Mine, Not Yours!"

"May you enjoy a childhood of rainbows, sunshine and happiness!"

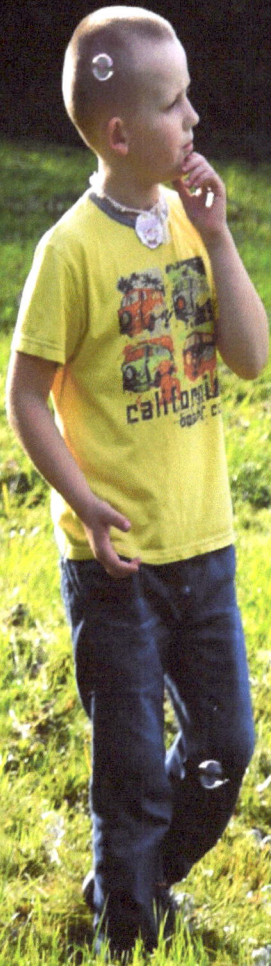

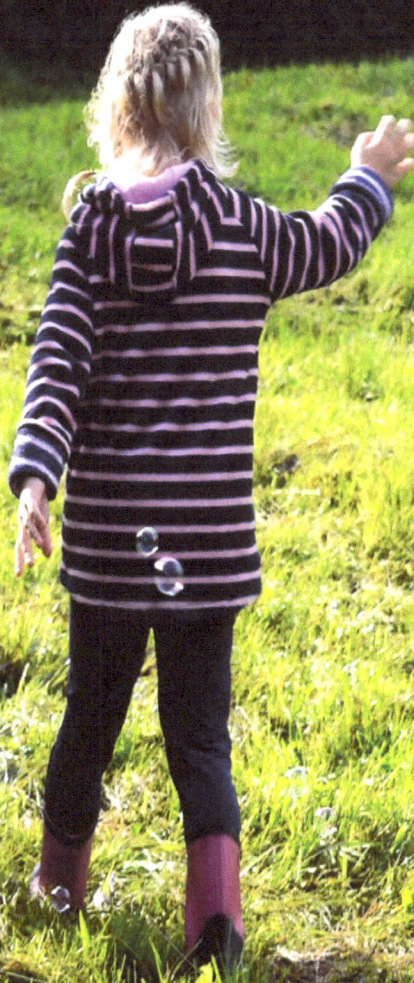

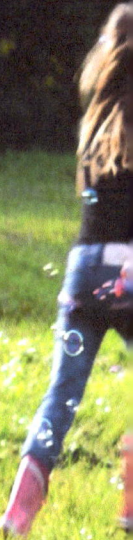

About the Author
Natalie Jane Lutter (N J Lutter)

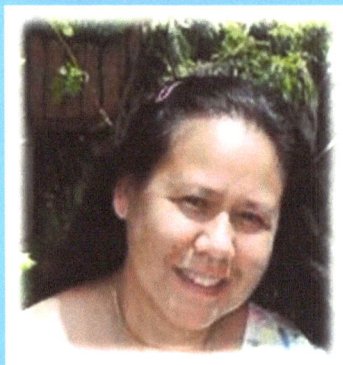

As Natalie knows only too well from her own experience as a child that the effect of Child Sexual Abuse is far reaching. Child Sexual Abuse can have a ripple effect on ones' life infiltrating many parts of a persons' life causing lifelong emotional problems, affecting relationships, self-esteem issues subsequently inflicting many emotional and physical disorders, depression and suicide. It has been of paramount importance to her to get her message out that children can be protected from Child Sexual Abuse.

Natalie lives on beautiful Macleay Island Qld Australia with her partner. She watched with pride her daughter grow and become a successful environmental scientist-her biggest joy in life! Natalie is a vocalist and author of self-help books namely "Conquering Cancer Fears," "Absolutely No Excuse For Abuse" with Companion Action Planner Journal and "Breaking the Chain on Abuse". She also keeps busy tending her garden to hold charity high teas and does guest speaking spots. Her interests are philanthropy and she is an advocate of many different charities, particularly humanities. She decided to write this book to help others as she is a survivor of child sexual abuse. It is her hope that by writing, "My Body Is Mine, Not Yours!" (Part 2) and accompanying book "The 3 E's Caregivers and Educators Companion Instructional Guide" (Part 1) she can help bring about prevention and awareness of child sexual abuse.

You can follow Natalie on Tumblr, Facebook, Twitter, Pinterest and Instagram or via www.globalselfhelptools.com

www.ingramcontent.com/pod-product-compliance
Lightning Source LLC
LaVergne TN
LVHW072119070426
835511LV00002B/19

9781925792300